Pediatric Otolaryngology: Challenges in Multi-system Disease

Guest Editor

AUSTIN S. ROSE, MD

OTOLARYNGOLOGIC CLINICS OF NORTH AMERICA

www.oto.theclinics.com

June 2012 • Volume 45 • Number 3

SAUNDERS an imprint of ELSEVIER, Inc.

W.B. SAUNDERS COMPANY
A Division of Elsevier Inc.

1600 John F. Kennedy Boulevard • Suite 1800 • Philadelphia, Pennsylvania 19103-2899

http://www.theclinics.com

OTOLARYNGOLOGIC CLINICS OF NORTH AMERICA Volume 45, Number 3
June 2012 ISSN 0030-6665, ISBN-13: 978-1-4557-3907-3

Editor: Joanne Husovski
Development Editor: Donald Mumford

Otolaryngologic Clinics of North America (ISSN 0030-6665) is published bimonthly by Elsevier, Inc., 360 Park Avenue South, New York, NY 10010-1710. Months of issue are February, April, June, August, October, and December. Business and Editorial Offices: 1600 John F. Kennedy Blvd., Suite 1800, Philadelphia, PA 19103-2899. Customer Service Office: 6277 Sea Harbor Drive, Orlando, FL 32887-4800. Periodicals postage paid at New York, NY and additional mailing offices. Subscription prices are $335.00 per year (US individuals), $628.00 per year (US institutions), $161.00 per year (US student/resident), $442.00 per year (Canadian individuals), $789.00 per year (Canadian institutions), $496.00 per year (international individuals), $789.00 per year (international institutions), $248.00 per year (international & Canadian student/resident). Foreign air speed delivery is included in all *Clinics*' subscription prices. All prices are subject to change without notice. **POSTMASTER:** Send address changes to *Otolaryngologic Clinics of North America*, Elsevier Health Sciences Division, Subscription Customer Service, 3251 Riverport Lane, Maryland Heights, MO 63043. **Telephone: 1-800-654-2452 (U.S. and Canada); 314-447-8871 (outside U.S. and Canada). Fax: 314-447-8029. E-mail: journalscustomerservice-usa@elsevier.com (for print support); journalsonlinesupport-usa@elsevier.com (for online support).**

Reprints. For copies of 100 or more of articles in this publication, please contact the Commercial Reprints Department, Elsevier Inc., 360 Park Avenue South, New York, NY 10010-1710. Tel.: 212-633-3812; Fax: 212-462-1935; E-mail: reprints@elsevier.com.

Otolaryngologic Clinics of North America is also published in Spanish by McGraw-Hill Interamericana Editores S.A., P.O. Box 5-237, 06500 Mexico D.F., Mexico.

Otolaryngologic Clinics of North America is covered in *MEDLINE/PubMed (Index Medicus), Current Contents/Clinical Medicine, Excerpta Medica, BIOSIS, Science Citation Index,* and *ISI/BIOMED.*

Printed and bound by CPI Group (UK) Ltd, Croydon, CR0 4YY

Transferred to Digital Print 2012

Contributors

GUEST EDITOR

AUSTIN S. ROSE, MD
Director, Pediatric Otolaryngology Fellowship Program; Associate Professor, Department of Otolaryngology–Head and Neck Surgery, University of North Carolina School of Medicine, Chapel Hill, North Carolina

AUTHORS

LISA M. BUCKMILLER, MD
Associate Professor, Pediatric Otolaryngology, Arkansas Children's Hospital, University of Arkansas for Medical Sciences, Little Rock, Arkansas

NADIESKA CABALLERO, MD
Resident, Division of Neurosciences, Department of Otolaryngology–Head and Neck Surgery, Stritch School of Medicine, Loyola University Hospital, Maywood, Illinois

AMELIA F. DRAKE, MD
Professor, Department of Otolaryngology–Head and Neck Surgery, University of North Carolina Hospital, Chapel Hill, North Carolina

CHARLES S. EBERT Jr, MD, MPH
Assistant Professor, Division of Rhinology, Allergy, and Endoscopic Skull Base Surgery, Department of Otolaryngology-Head and Neck Surgery, University of North Carolina School of Medicine, Chapel Hill, North Carolina

LARRY D. HARTZELL, MD
Instructor, Pediatric Otolaryngology Fellow, Arkansas Children's Hospital, University of Arkansas for Medical Sciences, Little Rock, Arkansas

JULIE HOOVER-FONG, MD, PhD
Alan and Kathryn Greenberg Center for Skeletal Dysplasias, McKusick-Nathans Institute of Genetic Medicine; Department of Pediatrics, Johns Hopkins University School of Medicine, Baltimore, Maryland

PAUL KRAKOVITZ, MD
Assistant Professor of Surgery, Section Head, Pediatric Otolaryngology, Head and Neck Institute, Cleveland Clinic, Cleveland, Ohio

SOFIA LYFORD-PIKE, MD
Department of Otolaryngology-Head and Neck Surgery, Johns Hopkins University School of Medicine, Baltimore, Maryland

KIBWEI A. MCKINNEY, MD
Resident Physician, Department of Otolaryngology-Head and Neck Surgery, University of North Carolina School of Medicine, Chapel Hill, North Carolina

JEREMY D. MEIER, MD
Assistant Professor, Division of Otolaryngology – Head and Neck Surgery, Department of Surgery, University of Utah, Salt Lake City, Utah

CANDACE A. MITCHELL, BA
Department of Otolaryngology-Head & Neck Surgery, University of North Carolina School of Medicine, Chapel Hill, North Carolina

HAROLD S. PINE, MD, FAAP
Assistant Professor, Department of Otolaryngology, University of Texas Medical Branch, Galveston, Texas

REGINA RODMAN, MD
Department of Otolaryngology, University of Texas Medical Branch, Galveston, Texas

AUSTIN S. ROSE, MD
Director, Pediatric Otolaryngology Fellowship Program; Associate Professor, Department of Otolaryngology–Head and Neck Surgery, University of North Carolina School of Medicine, Chapel Hill, North Carolina

JAMES M. RUDA, MD
Department of Otolaryngology-Head and Neck Surgery, University of North Carolina, Chapel Hill, North Carolina

ANDREW R. SCOTT, MD
Assistant Professor of Otolaryngology and Pediatrics, Department of Otolaryngology – Head & Neck Surgery, Floating Hospital for Children – Tufts Medical Center, Tufts University School of Medicine, Boston, Massachusetts

JAMES D. SIDMAN, MD
Pediatric ENT Associates, Children's Specialty Center, Children's Hospitals and Clinics of Minnesota; Professor of Otolaryngology and Pediatrics, Department of Otolaryngology, University of Minnesota Medical School, University of Minnesota, Minneapolis, Minnesota

LAURA H. SWIBEL ROSENTHAL, MD
Assistant Professor, Division of Neurosciences, Department of Otolaryngology–Head and Neck Surgery, Stritch School of Medicine, Loyola University Hospital, Maywood, Illinois

BRIAN D. THORP, MD
Resident Physician, Department of Otolaryngology-Head and Neck Surgery, University of North Carolina School of Medicine, Chapel Hill, North Carolina

ROBERT J. TIBESAR, MD
Pediatric ENT Associates, Children's Specialty Center, Children's Hospitals and Clinics of Minnesota; Assistant Professor of Otolaryngology, Department of Otolaryngology, University of Minnesota Medical School, University of Minnesota, Minneapolis, Minnesota

DAVID E. TUNKEL, MD
Department of Otolaryngology-Head and Neck Surgery; Department of Pediatrics, Johns Hopkins University School of Medicine, Baltimore, Maryland

MICHAEL P. UNDERBRINK, MD
Department of Otolaryngology, University of Texas Medical Branch, Galveston, Texas

NAREN N. VENKATESAN, MD
Department of Otolaryngology, University of Texas Medical Branch, Galveston, Texas

DAVID R. WHITE, MD
Associate Professor, Director, Pediatric Otolaryngology, Department of Otolaryngology –
Head and Neck Surgery, Medical University of South Carolina, Charleston,
South Carolina

ADAM M. ZANATION, MD
Department of Otolaryngology-Head & Neck Surgery, University of North Carolina School
of Medicine, Chapel Hill, North Carolina

Contents

This article reviews the most current practice guidelines in the diagnosis and treatment of infantile hemangiomas. Several systemic conditions that can be associated with hemangiomas, such as PHACES syndrome, are also discussed. Propranolol has become an effective first-line treatment, and protocols for its use as well as its potential risks are outlined.

This review describes important aspects of the most commonly encountered craniofacial syndromes. The goal is to provide otolaryngologists and other health care providers with critical information necessary to manage these patients appropriately. The algorithm provided in this article should be helpful in guiding the treatment of craniofacial patients based on their unique otolaryngologic characteristics. The principles highlighted in the algorithm can be applied to other craniofacial syndromes not addressed here, including Pierre Robin sequence and Down syndrome.

This article reviews some of the otolaryngologic manifestations of skeletal dysplasias. Achondroplasia is discussed most comprehensively. Skeletal dysplasias are bone and cartilage disorders that disrupt the development of the long bones, craniofacial skeleton, and vertebral column, with the most notable characteristic being short stature. Children with skeletal dysplasias have various medical problems. These children often develop head and neck manifestations of their disorders. Hearing loss, middle ear disease, and respiratory difficulties are seen in these children. Otolaryngologists must be knowledgeable about these disorders to diagnose, treat, and appropriately refer children with skeletal dysplasias.

As more patients with Down syndrome are living into adulthood, attention has focused on health factors that affect the quality of the patient's life and their ability to reach full potential. Patients with Down syndrome have several morphologic abnormalities that predispose them to problems with the ear, nose, and throat, and appropriate treatment can have a significant impact on the quality of life of these patients. Otolaryngologists are likely to see many patients with Down syndrome throughout their careers. This article reviews the literature to provide information and recommendations regarding management of Down syndrome.

Allergic fungal sinusitis (AFS) is a subtype of eosinophilic chronic rhinosinusitis (CRS) characterized by type I hypersensitivity, nasal polyposis, characteristic computed tomography scan findings, eosinophilic mucus, and the presence of fungus on surgical specimens without evidence of tissue invasion. This refractory subtype of CRS is of the great interest in the pediatric population, given the relatively early age of onset and the difficulty in managing AFS through commercially available medical regimens. Almost universally, a diagnosis of AFS requires operative intervention. Postoperative adjuvant medical therapy is a mainstay in the treatment paradigm of pediatric AFS.

Laryngotracheal reconstruction can be technically challenging. Successfully managing the patient's medical comorbidities is essential. Children undergoing laryngotracheal reconstruction rarely present with isolated subglottic stenosis; many have associated multisystem disorders. Effectively managing the patient enables successful outcomes after airway reconstruction.

This article highlights the most common causes of velopharyngeal insufficiency (VPI), and discusses routine evaluation and treatment algorithms for the managment of VPI in children. VPI is a multifactorial condition that occurs commonly in syndromic and non-syndromic children. The most common features of VPI are audible hypernasal speech, facial grimacing, decreased speech intelligibility, nasal regurgitation, and nasal emission from failure to produce oronasal separation. Work-up of VPI typically involves radiologic and endoscopic testing performed with the assistance of a speech-language pathologist. Management of VPI involves initial speech therapy followed by operative repair with sphincter or pharyngeal flap pharyngoplasty, if needed.

Recurrent respiratory papillomatosis (RRP) is a rare, benign disease with no known cure. RRP is caused by infection of the upper aerodigestive tract with the human papillomavirus (HPV). Passage through the birth canal is thought to be the initial transmission event, but infection may occur in utero. HPV vaccines have helped to provide protection from cervical cancer; however, their role in the prevention of RRP is undetermined. Clinical presentation of initial symptoms of RRP may be subtle. RRP course varies, and current management focuses on surgical debulking of papillomatous lesions with or without concurrent adjuvant therapy.

OTOLARYNGOLOGIC CLINICS OF NORTH AMERICA

FORTHCOMING ISSUES

HPV-Associated Head and Neck Cancer
Sara Pai, MD, *Guest Editor*

Evidence-Based Clinical Practice in Otolaryngology
Timothy Smith, MD, *Guest Editor*

Complementary Medicine in Otolaryngology
John Maddalozzo, MD,
Edmund Pribitkin, MD, and
Michael Seidman, MD,
Guest Editors

RELATED INTEREST

Pediatric Clinics of North America, June 2011 (Volume 58, Issue 3)
Pediatric Sleep Medicine Update
Judith A. Owens, MD, MPH, Jodi A. Mindell, PhD, *Guest Editors*

DOWNLOAD
Free App!

Review Articles
THE CLINICS

NOW AVAILABLE FOR YOUR iPhone and iPad

Preface

Treating Common Disorders in Complex Children

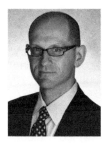

Austin S. Rose, MD
Guest Editor

Photo by Nicolette DeGroot, OHNS Communications UNC-Chapel Hill School of Medicine

One of the hallmarks in the current practice of pediatric otolaryngology is the treatment of common disorders in complex children. Whether the topic is airway management, sinusitis, or otologic disease, the skills and expertise of an experienced pediatric otolaryngologist can be of particular importance in the care of infants and children with congenital or genetic disorders, craniofacial syndromes, or other complex multi-system diseases. Yet the following articles are not intended solely for those within our relatively small field. It is my hope that our colleagues in a wide variety of practices, including pediatrics, general otolaryngology, and speech and language pathology, will also find this information helpful and, in some cases, invaluable.

Several of the articles do, in fact, specifically address common problems or procedures in more complicated children, such as those with Down syndrome, skeletal dysplasia, or a variety of craniofacial syndromes. Such children, whether due to unusual anatomy or underlying pathophysiology affecting multiple organ systems, can present particular challenges in management. Some of the most recent advances in pediatric otolaryngology are also covered in detail, including the significant changes in management for infantile hemangiomas. In addition, the increasing experience with endoscopic sinus surgery and skull-base techniques in pediatric patients is discussed. In particular, the role of these techniques in improving the care of children with allergic fungal sinusitis and juvenile nasopharyngeal angiofibroma is presented.

The layout of the articles is intended for the easiest possible access to important information. In addition to a summary of key points and highlighted *"Pearls & Pitfalls,"* a number of video links are presented with instructions to access these additional materials on-line. Some authors have provided notes that are especially helpful for pediatricians.

I would like to thank each of the authors for their time and contributions. Their work here reflects to a significant degree some of the most current knowledge in pediatric

Otolaryngol Clin N Am 45 (2012) xi–xii
doi:10.1016/j.otc.2012.03.011
0030-6665/12/$ – see front matter © 2012 Elsevier Inc. All rights reserved.

oto.theclinics.com

otolaryngology. I would also like to thank those who have inspired and guided my work in the field as well, including Drs Harold C. Pillsbury III, Amelia F. Drake, and Brent A. Senior here at the University of North Carolina, my fellowship director, Dr David E. Tunkel, at Johns Hopkins University in Baltimore, MD, and my tireless and always available partners within the Division of Rhinology, Allergy, and Sinus Surgery, Drs Charles S. Ebert Jr and Adam M. Zanation.

Austin S. Rose, MD
Pediatric Otolaryngology Fellowship Program

Department of Otolaryngology–Head and Neck Surgery
University of North Carolina School of Medicine
Campus Box #7070
Chapel Hill, NC 27599-7070, USA

E-mail address:
austin_rose@med.unc.edu

Current Management of Infantile Hemangiomas and Their Common Associated Conditions

Larry D. Hartzell, MD, Lisa M. Buckmiller, MD*

KEYWORDS

- Infantile hemangioma • Hemangioma • Hemangioma treatment • PHACES
- Propranolol

KEY POINTS

- Correct diagnosis of hemangioma is imperative for appropriate treatment.
- Be familiar with the current classification of all vascular anomalies.
- Infantile hemangiomas are benign with a defined clinical course, involution only occurring in infancy and never later.
- Large, obstructing, or ulcerative lesions require early treatment to prevent functional deficits, pain, and physical deformity.
- Physicians should be aware of syndromes/conditions that can be associated with hemangiomas.
- Propranolol has revolutionized how hemangiomas are treated, but caution should be exercised.

The most common tumors of infancy and early childhood are hemangiomas.[1] These tumors are benign, but their health implications can be severe. Although many of these lesions do not require treatment, a significant number require multiple treatments and may present therapeutic challenges. This notion deviates from the commonly held belief that such birthmarks should only be observed and will resolve with time.

Hemangiomas can present as focal or segmental lesions and superficial, deep, or compound in nature.[2] Although most hemangiomas are solitary lesions in uncomplicated locations, a significant number will present in locations with higher morbidity or as a component of a more systemic disease process. This review is intended to

Pediatric Otolaryngology, Arkansas Children's Hospital, University of Arkansas for Medical Sciences, 1 Children's Way, Slot 668, Little Rock, AR 72202, USA
* Corresponding author.
E-mail address: Buckmillerlisam@uams.edu

Otolaryngol Clin N Am 45 (2012) 545–556
doi:10.1016/j.otc.2012.03.001
0030-6665/12/$ – see front matter © 2012 Elsevier Inc. All rights reserved.

assist the practitioner with the diagnostic tools and therapeutic options that are essential in the proper management of these common yet sometimes challenging lesions.

DEMOGRAPHICS OF HEMANGIOMAS

Hemangiomas are found in 4% to 10% of all infants and in up to 30% of premature babies.[1,3,4] Sixty percent of hemangiomas are found in the head and neck region.[5] The most common predisposing factors for the development of a hemangioma are[3]:

- Caucasian ethnicity
- Female sex (71% female or 2.4:1 female-to-male ratio)
- Low birth weight
- Products of multiple gestations.

Advanced maternal age and the presence of placenta previa have also been shown to be significant factors.[3]

Many retrospective and prospective studies have focused on elucidating the reason for this specific demographic distribution, with very few answers.

ETIOLOGY OF HEMANGIOMAS

The inheritance of hemangiomas is mainly sporadic. However, in a study by Haggstrom and colleagues,[3] one-third of their patients with hemangiomas had a first-degree relative with a vascular lesion and 12% had a first-degree relative who had a hemangioma. Genetic research has discovered an association with chromosome 5, but this has only been discovered in a small percentage of patients.[6,7] Autosomal dominance has also been reported in some cases.[8]

Although the genetic factors are often uncertain, the basic nature of hemangiomas is becoming increasingly well understood. An active area of current hemangioma research is the molecular markers and growth factors associated with hemangiomas. In a landmark article, North and colleagues[9] described the presence of GLUT1, a glucose transporter typically limited to endothelium in tissues with a blood-tissue barrier, which was present in 97% of the juvenile hemangiomas studied. The investigators then discovered that GLUT1 was not present in any other vascular lesions including pyogenic granulomas, granulation tissue, and venous, lymphatic, or arteriovenous malformations. Further studies identified other markers such as FcγRII, merosin, and LeY, which are all present in hemangiomas as well as placental tissue while being spared in other body tissues.[10] The tissue architecture of hemangiomas is, however, different to that of placental tissue, which suggests a common progenitor cell or a shared regulatory mechanism.

A few hypotheses have been presented to explain the "hemangioma-placental connection."[10,11] These theories include somatic mutations, abnormal local inductive influences from the placenta, or placental emboli that were shed and received by the developing placental tissues. Of these, the embolic theory has found some support, as patients with chorionic villus sampling have been found to have an increased incidence of hemangiomas.[12]

CLASSIFICATION OF HEMANGIOMAS AMONG VASCULAR ANOMALIES

The distinction of hemangiomas from other vascular lesions is a critical area of understanding for any practitioner who may see these patients. Although hemangiomas are the most common vascular lesion, not all vascular lesions are hemangiomas, and each type of lesion will have its own specific clinical course.

In 1982, Mulliken and Glowacki[13] published a classification scheme that has been used as the primer for the current internationally accepted nomenclature and distinction of vascular lesions. This classification separated vascular anomalies into 2 major categories: (1) vascular tumors and (2) vascular malformations.

Vascular tumors grow through endothelial proliferation and have the potential for spontaneous regression. Vascular malformations, however, grow via vessel ectasia and will not resolve with time. A thorough description of each subclassification of vascular anomalies and their individual clinical course is beyond the scope of this article, and it is strongly recommended that the reader refer to the original document for further enlightenment.

Among the vascular tumors group, the dominant member is hemangiomas. Within the hemangioma category of vascular lesions, there are also different subtypes.

Infantile Hemangiomas

Hemangiomas that are not identified at birth or are very small and then progressively grow are called infantile hemangiomas. These hemangiomas follow a proliferative growth phase followed by quiescence and involution, and are the focus of this review.
Infantile hemangiomas can be:

- Focal or segmental
- Superficial or deep
- Single or diffuse.

These factors can help the practitioner with risk stratification and may provide a clue to a more systemic process.[14,15]

Congenital Hemangiomas

Those hemangiomas that are fully developed at birth and do not undergo more than proportional postnatal growth are called congenital hemangiomas.[16] These lesions are rare and have an incidence of about 3% of all hemangiomas.[9] Histologically they are different from infantile hemangiomas.[17] Within the congenital hemangioma category, there are also 2 subtypes[18,19]:

1. Noninvoluting congenital hemangioma (NICH).
2. Rapidly involuting congenital hemangioma (RICH).

CLINICAL COURSE OF HEMANGIOMAS

Infantile hemangiomas are vascular tumors that grow intermittently throughout the first year of life. The majority achieve up to two-thirds of their size during the first 5 months of life.[20] Some infantile hemangiomas are visibly present at birth and others are noticed later, depending on depth and extent. Close observation and early subspecialist referral should be considered during this early growth phase.

The growth of infantile hemangiomas proceeds through different phases: the proliferative phase continues usually throughout the first 9 to 12 months of life followed by quiescence, which is of variable length, and then involution, which may last several years.

Proliferative Phase

During the proliferative phase of an infantile hemangioma, it is important for the practitioner to monitor the patient closely. It is typically during this phase that early treatment is considered if significant growth is occurring, ulceration results, or functional consequences are developing. Ulceration is common in rapidly growing lesions that have a superficial component. Such lesions can cause significant pain, bleeding, and excessive scarring if they are not recognized and treated early.

Quiescence/Involution

Once the rapid growth phase tapers off the involuting phase commences, which includes the stabilization of the size of the tumor and commencement of regression. Practically all infantile hemangiomas eventually involute, but the timing of involution and extent of hemangioma regression can be highly variable. The earliest signs of involution commonly include a graying of the lesion centrally and often a subtle, diffuse darkening of the lesion. This phase is typically the longest, with completion of involution taking from 1 to 7 years.[16] Once a hemangioma has entered the involution phase it never regrows, which helps distinguish hemangiomas from vascular malformations.

Involuted Phase

The final presentation of the infantile hemangioma is the involuted phase. The involuted hemangioma is typically found to have overlying atrophic skin and excessive fibrofatty tissue with overlying telangiectasias.

SPECIAL CONSIDERATIONS IN HEMANGIOMAS
Beard-Distribution Hemangiomas

Beard-distribution hemangiomas involve the V3 distribution of the trigeminal nerve. These patients have segmental superficial hemangiomas along preauricular and mandibular distribution including the lower lip, as well as airway involvement. These patients also frequently have hemangioma involvement of both parotid glands. Most importantly, patients with beard-distribution hemangiomas commonly have airway involvement, typically in the subglottis. Airway hemangiomas occur in about 65% of beard-distribution hemangiomas and are frequently not symptomatic until the fourth to eighth week of life when hemangioma growth is most rapid.[21] It is recommended that all patients, when diagnosed with a beard-distribution hemangioma, undergo diagnostic microlaryngoscopy and bronchoscopy to ascertain the presence of airway involvement. It should also be noted that hemangioma can occur anywhere in the airway, but subglottic involvement is usually the most problematic (**Fig. 1**).

PHACES Syndrome

Segmental superficial hemangiomas in the head and neck should alert the physician to the possibility of PHACES syndrome; this is especially true if the hemangioma is in the V1, V2, or scalp distribution. PHACES syndrome can represent abnormalities in[22]:

Posterior cranial fossa (frequently cerebellum)
Hemangiomas of the face/scalp
Arterial abnormalities
Cardiac abnormalities
Eye abnormalities
Sternal clefting (or umbilical raphe).

Patients with segmental hemangiomas of the face/scalp need to have further diagnostic studies to rule out other abnormalities. A careful physical examination, looking for outward defects such as ocular hemangioma/strabismus as well as sternal or

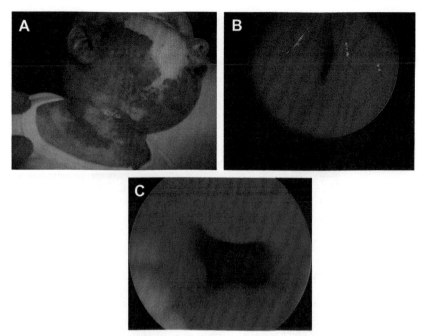

Fig. 1. (A) A 2-month-old infant with beard-distribution hemangioma. (B) Bilateral subglottic involvement in another patient with beard-distribution hemangioma. (C) Tracheal involvement in patient shown in B.

umbilical raphe, should be performed. Diagnostic studies that should be obtained include:

- Magnetic resonance imaging (MRI)/magnetic resonance angiography of the brain/face/neck to look for intracranial and arterial abnormalities
- Echocardiogram to examine the cardiac structures
- Ophthalmologic examination (**Fig. 2**).

Systemic Hemangiomatosis

Patients with multiple external hemangiomas (more than 4 or 5) should be examined for intra-abdominal involvement. The most common organ involved in these patients is the liver, and thus the first study of choice is abdominal ultrasonography. If hemangiomas are suspected or identified on ultrasound examination, an MRI should be performed to further define the extent (**Fig. 3**). Patients with extensive liver or intra-abdominal involvement need immediate treatment, as liver failure and consumptive hypothyroidism can result.[23,24]

Sacral Hemangiomas

Hemangiomas overlying the sacrum and lumbar spine should alert the practitioner to potential spinal cord abnormalities such as spina bifida or, more commonly, tethered cord. If the child is younger than 3 months, an ultrasound examination can typically rule out such abnormalities. Otherwise, an MRI of the lower spine is recommended.

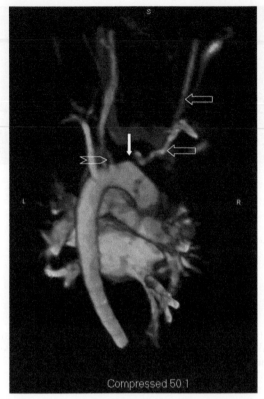

Fig. 2. MRA in PHACES patient. Note the near complete stenosis of the brachiocephalic artery (*filled arrow*), filling of the right brachiocephalic and carotid arteries from the right vertebral artery (*hollow arrows*), and the left vertebral artery branching directly from the aortic arch (*arrowhead*).

TREATMENT OF HEMANGIOMAS

The treatment of infantile hemangiomas is always individualized to the specific lesion as well as to the patient. There are many options for treatment, and it is essential to

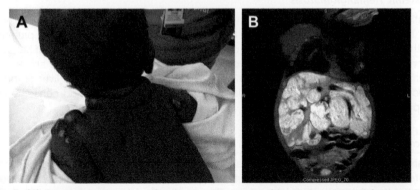

Fig. 3. (*A*) External appearance of patient with systemic hemangiomatosis. (*B*) Near total liver replacement with hemangioma in patient shown in *A*.

have a thorough knowledge of these differing treatment modalities to properly counsel the family. In many cases treatment is elective, with more than one "right choice."

The timing and type of intervention selected needs to be tailored to the specific patient and hemangioma in question. It is also important that infantile hemangiomas will not always respond to the same treatment. Moreover, some infantile hemangiomas are difficult to differentiate from congenital hemangiomas and, more importantly, from more aggressive tumors (such as arteriovenous malformations, tufted angiomas, fibrosarcomas, and rhabdomyosarcomas). In these cases, early biopsy or excision may be indicated.

Infantile hemangiomas can require a complicated treatment algorithm. Much of the decision making involves location, growth history, size, and complications. It is the location and extent of the lesion that will frequently drive intervention. Single small lesions or small superficial lesions are less likely to require intervention than large, bulky, or multiple lesions to require intervention. Several areas demand special attention, because hemangiomas in these areas can result in an increased incidence of morbidity or enhanced consequences of the associated deformity. These areas include the periorbital region, the nasal tip, the paranasal region, and the subglottis, among others, and will often require treatment.

Observation

As previously mentioned, observation is frequently selected in the majority of infantile hemangiomas especially if the hemangioma is early in the proliferation phase. Observation allows time to help distinguish an infantile hemangioma from another type of lesion, and may help determine which lesions will result in functional or cosmetic deformity. Close follow-up is recommended in this period in case any complications do arise that may necessitate early treatment. Early intervention should be pursued in some hemangiomas, depending on growth rate, extent, location, and complications.

Medical Management

For many patients with hemangiomas, nonsurgical methods are considered early, during the proliferative phase. Corticosteroids have been considered the standard medical treatment through the years. However, in the past few years β-blockers have become a first-line treatment for many hemangiomas. Other pharmacologic therapies are available for resistant or complicated lesions, but such cases are rare.

Propranolol for Hemangiomas

In 2008, Leaute-Labreze and colleagues[25] reported in an editorial of the *New England Journal of Medicine* about the serendipitous discovery of the beneficial effect of the nonselective β-blocker, propranolol, on the growth of hemangiomas. This report, and its follow-up report in 2009,[26] set in motion a flurry of research and clinical applications that has revolutionized the management of hemangiomas. Although the exact mechanism of propranolol on hemangiomas is not known, it has been suggested that it may gain its efficacy through mechanisms of vasoconstriction or apoptosis. These mechanisms are areas of active investigation in many institutions.

Propranolol is now considered the first-line therapy for many hemangiomas.[27] Common side effects of this medication are hypersomnolence, increased gastroesophageal reflux and, less commonly, night terrors, bronchospasm, hypoglycemia, and growth disturbance. In general, propranolol has been found to be well tolerated by most patients, with an overall side effect profile less problematic than that of oral steroids. A thorough initial workup along with the involvement of a pediatric cardiologist is strongly recommended (**Box 1**).

> **Box 1**
> **Propranolol protocol**
>
> - Thorough history (cardiopulmonary, diabetes, reflux) including family history
> - Tests: electrocardiogram (echocardiography if positive history), glucose, vitals + weight
> - Consent for off-label use
> - Cardiologist clearance
> - Dose: 2 mg/kg divided TID (follow-up with PCP in 48–72 hours for vitals and glucose check)
> - RTC at 1 month for weight check and side effects
> - RTC every 3 months until treatment is finished (usually until 1 year of age)
> - Cessation: cut dose in half for 1 week and then stop
> - RTC at 3 months for reevaluation
>
> *Abbreviations:* PCP, primary care physician; RTC, return to clinic; TID, 3 times per day.

To date, the use of propranolol for hemangiomas is off-label, and families should be counseled accordingly. No prospective randomized trials using propranolol have been published to date and its use is still considered investigational, therefore caution must be exercised regarding its use.

The degree of propranolol efficacy reported in the literature is variable. In a study by Buckmiller and colleagues,[28] performed at the authors' institution, 97% of patients were found to be at least partial responders to this medication with 50% falling into the excellent-response group. Minor side effects were encountered in about one-third of patients but were easily managed. With a multitude of current literature supporting the efficacy and safety of the novel application of this established medication, propranolol should be a consideration when the management of any hemangioma is being addressed.

Corticosteroids for Hemangiomas

Systemic corticosteroids were the mainstay in the pharmacologic management of infantile hemangiomas since the 1960s, when its beneficial effects were incidentally discovered by Zarem and Edgerton.[29] Steroids have proved to be effective in controlling and even reversing the growth of proliferating hemangiomas. However, significant side effects (such as growth disturbance, adrenal suppression, hypertension, and behavioral changes) are frequently encountered.[30,31] In addition, the beneficial effects of systemic corticosteroids are not permanent, and rebound growth of the hemangioma frequently occurs after cessation of the medication. Because of this, systemic steroids have had their first-line treatment status changed by most practitioners. Its indications are now mainly in short-term management, such as in acute respiratory distress from an airway lesion.

Injected corticosteroids (such as triamcinolone) also serve an important role in the management of hemangiomas. One benefit of this method is the limitation of the systemic effects of corticosteroids. However, in some areas (ie, periocular), the injection method presents a serious risk of corticosteroid particle embolization, which can have serious consequences.[32,33] Nevertheless, when properly selected and carefully applied, steroid injection can be a valuable tool in the management of focal hemangiomas.

Vincristine for Hemangiomas

Vincristine, a chemotherapeutic agent, was identified as a better alternative to the potentially disabling interferon-α treatment. Its use is largely reserved for individuals with kaposiform hemangioendothelioma that progresses to Kasabach-Merritt syndrome, or in extensive hemangiomatosis not responsive to other treatments.[34,35] The side effects are typically limited and tolerable. Because of its increased safety profile, vincristine is the preferred medication for these isolated, complex cases. Management of these patients by a specialized hematologist/oncologist is recommended.

Interferon for Hemangiomas

Interferon-α2a, an antiviral agent, was established as an effective medication to treat steroid-resistant hemangiomas.[36–38] However, despite the good response to treatment, serious side effects may transpire with the use of this drug. Most notable among these is irreversible spastic diplegia. Because of this, and the availability of other equally or more effective medications such as vincristine, this agent is not currently recommended unless it is the only alternative in a life-threatening situation.

Laser Therapy for Hemangiomas

One of the mainstay therapies for infantile hemangiomas is laser photocoagulation. The most common and effective laser for hemangioma treatment is the pulsed dye laser (PDL).[39] With a wavelength of 595 nm, PDL is preferentially absorbed by the chromophore oxyhemoglobin, which is found abundantly in superficial hemangiomas. This modality can be used early on to assist with ulceration treatment and prevention.[40] It is also more frequently used later during the involution or involuted phases to reduce or eliminate telangiectasias or residual staining. It has been shown that the early use of PDL also has a beneficial effect on the final scar and textural quality of the residual affected skin, with a low incidence of complications.[41]

Surgery for Hemangiomas

With the use of current medication options such as propranolol, as well as laser photocoagulation, the number of patients requiring surgical excision has been decreasing. Early surgical intervention may occasionally be considered in patients who have hemangiomas causing significant morbidity (ie, persistent ulceration, symptomatic and unresponsive subglottic or periorbital hemangioma, and so forth). In other patients, surgery may be considered once the proliferative phase has passed and involution has commenced or completed. Patients who will benefit from late excision are frequently those with persistent bulk causing tissue deformity. Large, compound hemangiomas end up behaving like tissue expanders, and significant asymmetry or functional impairment can result.

Patients who will benefit from surgical excision are generally identified in the first few years of life, and treatment is offered early to take advantage of the remarkable healing capacity of young children. Most surgeons will recommend treatment before the school-age years, to minimize the social impact of these potentially deforming lesions.

When surgery is pursued, several principles are followed. First, not all hemangioma tissue needs to be excised. In small lesions complete excision is appropriate. However, it is important to recognize that residual hemangioma will become fibrofatty tissue with time and will thus provide the appropriate bulk to the subcutaneous tissue that native tissues would have accomplished. One should never consider complete excision in extensive lesions, as the resultant deformity would be unacceptable. Second, the principles of reconstruction with careful consideration of relaxed skin-tension lines and the minimization of scarring should also be observed. Third, lasers can be a useful adjunct to surgical excision for treatment of any remaining discoloration with PDL or to improve atrophic scarring with laser resurfacing.

SUMMARY

Hemangiomas are the most common benign tumor of infancy, and the vast majority present in the head and neck. Therefore, it is important for the practicing physician to be aware of treatment options as well as the associated abnormalities that may accompany these lesions. Watchful waiting may be indicated in small uncomplicated hemangiomas; however, in larger lesions that are more likely to cause disfigurement or functional problems, intervention is recommended. The last several years have witnessed a paradigm shift in the treatment of these lesions with the application of propranolol. Although it is widely used and outstanding results have been seen with the its use, propranolol is not appropriate for all patients, and caution is strongly advised.

REFERENCES

1. Jacobs AH, Walton RG. The incidence of birthmarks in the neonate. Pediatrics 1976;58:218–22.
2. Chiller KG, Passaro D, Frieden IJ. Hemangiomas of infancy: clinical characteristics, morphologic subtypes, and their relationship to race, ethnicity, and sex. Arch Dermatol 2002;138:1567–76.
3. Haggstrom AN, Drolet BA, Baselga E, et al. Prospective study of infantile hemangiomas: demographic, prenatal, and perinatal characteristics. J Pediatr 2007; 150:291–4.
4. Smolinski KN, Yan AC. Hemangiomas of infancy: clinical and biological characteristics. Clin Pediatr (Phila) 2005;44:747–66.
5. Macarthur CJ. Head and neck hemangiomas of infancy. Curr Opin Otolaryngol Head Neck Surg 2006;14:397–405.
6. Berg JN, Walter JW, Thisanagayam U, et al. Evidence for loss of heterozygosity of 5q in sporadic haemangiomas: are somatic mutations involved in haemangioma formation? J Clin Pathol 2001;54:249–52.
7. Walter JW, Blei F, Anderson JL, et al. Genetic mapping of a novel familial form of infantile hemangioma. Am J Med Genet 1999;82:77–83.
8. Blei F, Walter J, Orlow SJ, et al. Familial segregation of hemangiomas and vascular malformations as an autosomal dominant trait. Arch Dermatol 1998; 134:718–22.
9. North PE, Waner M, Mizeracki A, et al. GLUT1: a newly discovered immunohistochemical marker for juvenile hemangiomas. Hum Pathol 2000;31:11–22.
10. North PE, Waner M, Mizeracki A, et al. A unique microvascular phenotype shared by juvenile hemangiomas and human placenta. Arch Dermatol 2001;137:559–70.
11. North PE, Waner M, Brodsky MC. Are infantile hemangiomas of placental origin? Ophthalmology 2002;109:633–4.
12. Burton BK, Schulz CJ, Angle B, et al. An increased incidence of haemangiomas in infants born following chorionic villus sampling (CVS). Prenat Diagn 1995;15: 209–14.
13. Mulliken JB, Glowacki J. Classification of pediatric vascular lesions. Plast Reconstr Surg 1982;70:120–1.
14. Haggstrom AN, Lammer EJ, Schneider RA, et al. Patterns of infantile hemangiomas: new clues to hemangioma pathogenesis and embryonic facial development. Pediatrics 2006;117:698–703.
15. Waner M, North PE, Scherer KA, et al. The nonrandom distribution of facial hemangiomas. Arch Dermatol 2003;139:869–75.

16. Mulliken JB, Enjolras O. Congenital hemangiomas and infantile hemangioma: missing links. J Am Acad Dermatol 2004;50:875–82.
17. Berenguer B, Mulliken JB, Enjolras O, et al. Rapidly involuting congenital hemangioma: clinical and histopathologic features. Pediatr Dev Pathol 2003;6:495–510.
18. Krol A, MacArthur CJ. Congenital hemangiomas: rapidly involuting and noninvoluting congenital hemangiomas. Arch Facial Plast Surg 2005;7:307–11.
19. Enjolras O, Mulliken JB, Boon LM, et al. Noninvoluting congenital hemangioma: a rare cutaneous vascular anomaly. Plast Reconstr Surg 2001;107:1647–54.
20. Chang LC, Haggstrom AN, Drolet BA, et al. Growth characteristics of infantile hemangiomas: implications for management. Pediatrics 2008;122:360–7.
21. Orlow SJ, Isakoff MS, Blei F. Increased risk of symptomatic hemangiomas of the airway in association with cutaneous hemangiomas in a "beard" distribution. J Pediatr 1997;131:643–6.
22. Roganovic J, Adams D. PHACES syndrome—case report and literature review. Coll Antropol 2009;33:311–4.
23. Cho YH, Taplin C, Mansour A, et al. Case report: consumptive hypothyroidism consequent to multiple infantile hepatic haemangiomas. Curr Opin Pediatr 2008;20:213–5.
24. Peters C, Langham S, Mullis PE, et al. Use of combined liothyronine and thyroxine therapy for consumptive hypothyroidism associated with hepatic haemangiomas in infancy. Horm Res Paediatr 2010;74:149–52.
25. Leaute-Labreze C, Dumas de la Roque E, Hubiche T, et al. Propranolol for severe hemangiomas of infancy. N Engl J Med 2008;358:2649–51.
26. Sans V, de la Roque ED, Berge J, et al. Propranolol for severe infantile hemangiomas: follow-up report. Pediatrics 2009;124:e423–31.
27. Fuchsmann C, Quintal MC, Giguere C, et al. Propranolol as first-line treatment of head and neck hemangiomas. Arch Otolaryngol Head Neck Surg 2011;137: 471–8.
28. Buckmiller LM, Munson PD, Dyamenahalli U, et al. Propranolol for infantile hemangiomas: early experience at a tertiary vascular anomalies center. Laryngoscope 2010;120:676–81.
29. Zarem HA, Edgerton MT. Induced resolution of cavernous hemangiomas following prednisolone therapy. Plast Reconstr Surg 1967;39:76–83.
30. Sadan N, Wolach B. Treatment of hemangiomas of infants with high doses of prednisone. J Pediatr 1996;128:141–6.
31. Boon LM, MacDonald DM, Mulliken JB. Complications of systemic corticosteroid therapy for problematic hemangioma. Plast Reconstr Surg 1999;104:1616–23.
32. Shorr N, Seiff SR. Central retinal artery occlusion associated with periocular corticosteroid injection for juvenile hemangioma. Ophthalmic Surg 1986;17:229–31.
33. Ruttum MS, Abrams GW, Harris GJ, et al. Bilateral retinal embolization associated with intralesional corticosteroid injection for capillary hemangioma of infancy. J Pediatr Ophthalmol Strabismus 1993;30:4–7.
34. Boehm DK, Kobrinsky NL. Treatment of cavernous hemangioma with vincristine. Ann Pharmacother 1993;27:981.
35. Perez Payarols J, Pardo Masferrer J, Gomez Bellvert C. Treatment of life-threatening infantile hemangiomas with vincristine. N Engl J Med 1995;333:69.
36. Ezekowitz RA, Mulliken JB, Folkman J. Interferon alfa-2a therapy for life-threatening hemangiomas of infancy. N Engl J Med 1992;326:1456–63.
37. Ricketts RR, Hatley RM, Corden BJ, et al. Interferon-alpha-2a for the treatment of complex hemangiomas of infancy and childhood. Ann Surg 1994;219:605–12 [discussion: 12–4].

38. Chang E, Boyd A, Nelson CC, et al. Successful treatment of infantile hemangiomas with interferon-alpha-2b. J Pediatr Hematol Oncol 1997;19:237–44.
39. Shafirstein G, Buckmiller LM, Waner M, et al. Mathematical modeling of selective photothermolysis to aid the treatment of vascular malformations and hemangioma with pulsed dye laser. Lasers Med Sci 2007;22:111–8.
40. Thomas RF, Hornung RL, Manning SC, et al. Hemangiomas of infancy: treatment of ulceration in the head and neck. Arch Facial Plast Surg 2005;7:312–5.
41. Hohenleutner S, Badur-Ganter E, Landthaler M, et al. Long-term results in the treatment of childhood hemangioma with the flashlamp-pumped pulsed dye laser: an evaluation of 617 cases. Lasers Surg Med 2001;28:273–7.

Otolaryngologic Manifestations of Craniofacial Syndromes

Laura H. Swibel Rosenthal, MD[a],*, Nadieska Caballero, MD[a],
Amelia F. Drake, MD[b]

KEYWORDS

- Craniofacial • Apert syndrome • Crouzon syndrome • Treacher Collins syndrome
- DiGeorge syndrome • Velocardiofacial syndrome • Opitz G/BBB syndrome
- Moebius syndrome

KEY POINTS

- A multidisciplinary approach is paramount in the management of the craniofacial patient.
- The first step in management of this patient population is ensuring a safe airway.
- Nasal obstruction and obstructive sleep apnea are serious potential problems in this patient population.
- Evaluation of most craniofacial patients should include a flexible nasopharyngoscopy that can identify choanal atresia, submucous clefts, velopharyngeal insufficiency, nasopharyngeal depth, vocal cord function, and laryngeal clefts and webs.
- A conservative approach is needed in patients with cleft palate or submucous cleft when performing an adenoidectomy, as it can lead to velopharyngeal insufficiency.
- Craniofacial patients typically require multiple corrective surgeries, performed in staged fashion, requiring computed tomography scan and/or magnetic resonance imaging in preoperative planning.
- It is essential to consider and address:
  - Hearing loss
  - Otitis media
  - Social and psychological implications of craniofacial abnormalities
  - Challenges with endotracheal intubation and mask ventilation
  - Presence of aspiration and gastroesophageal reflux.

Funding support: None.
Financial disclosures, conflicts of interest: The authors have nothing to disclose.
[a] Division of Neurosciences, Department of Otolaryngology – Head and Neck Surgery, Stritch School of Medicine, Loyola University Hospital, 2160 South First Avenue, Maywood, IL 60153-5500, USA; [b] Department of Otolaryngology – Head and Neck Surgery, University of North Carolina Hospital, Physician Office Building, CB#7070, 101 Manning Drive, Chapel Hill, NC 27514, USA
* Corresponding author.
E-mail address: LHRosenthal@lumc.edu

doi:10.1016/j.otc.2012.03.009
oto.theclinics.com

The management of patients with craniofacial syndromes is complex. Otolaryngologic evaluation is of paramount importance in providing adequate care for this patient population because patients commonly have airway, feeding, speech, and hearing problems. This review describes important aspects of the most commonly encountered craniofacial syndromes. In addition, the authors aim to provide otolaryngologists and other health care providers with critical information necessary to manage these patients appropriately.

The algorithm provided in this article should be helpful in guiding the treatment of craniofacial patients based on their unique otolaryngologic characteristics. Many aspects of care for this patient population are the same, regardless of the disease process. The principles highlighted in the algorithm can be applied to other craniofacial syndromes not addressed here, including Pierre Robin sequence and Down syndrome, discussed in articles elsewhere in this issue.

GENERAL CONCEPTS IN MANAGEMENT
Airway

In otolaryngology, the first step in managing a patient with a craniofacial syndrome is ensuring that he or she has a safe airway; this may start with positioning or other supportive measures. However, some patients require a surgical airway. In one craniofacial clinic, nearly 20% of the 251 craniofacial patients enrolled required a tracheotomy.[1] Most patients will have a flexible and/or direct laryngoscopy. Addressing the airway often involves ruling out aspiration and treating it appropriately if present. Workup often includes a video swallow and esophagram. Evaluation of speech pathology is important, first for feeding and later for speech and language development.

> PEARLS & PITFALLS: *The first step in managing a patient with craniofacial syndromes is to ensure a safe airway. In addition, the otolaryngologist must be aware of the great potential for nasal obstruction and sleep apnea in craniofacial patients.*

Gastrointestinal Problems

Gastrointestinal congenital anomalies or common problems such as reflux should be treated. The otolaryngologist must be aware of the great potential for nasal obstruction and sleep apnea in craniofacial patients. In addition, craniofacial patients have a higher risk of developing common otolaryngologic diseases, including upper airway problems such as rhinitis, sinusitis, or laryngitis.

Hearing Loss

Another common problem in this patient population is hearing loss. In addition to the newborn hearing screen performed in the United States, craniofacial patients need to continue to be followed with serial audiograms because hearing loss is common and may be progressive. Those with chronic otitis media may require tympanostomy tubes. Other causes of hearing loss may necessitate surgical intervention as well. However, assistive hearing devices are recommended for many patients, starting early in life.

Multidisciplinary Approach

A multidisciplinary team approach is paramount in the management of the craniofacial patient population. Patients should undergo a genetic workup to determine the etiology of the malformation and identify other potential associated medical problems. Furthermore, genetic counseling can help provide parents with reasonable expectations related to the care of the patient and help them understand potential implications for other family members. In addition to otolaryngologists, pulmonologists and gastroenterologists also commonly provide care for craniofacial patients. Dentists and orthodontists play a crucial role. Most patients need additional support services, such as case management (social work), psychology or psychiatry, speech pathology, physical therapy, occupational therapy, and other educational services. Because of congenital anomalies associated with specific syndromes, various other pediatric specialists may need to be consulted, including cardiologists, ophthalmologists, neurosurgeons, endocrinologists, urologists, nephrologists, and orthopedic surgeons.

Surgical Anesthesia Challenges

Patients with craniofacial syndromes may require multiple surgeries. Surgeons and anesthesiologists should be aware of the potential challenges these patients may have with general anesthesia.[2] In particular, endotracheal intubation or even mask ventilation may be difficult. Patients with micrognathia or macroglossia may be difficult to intubate. Patients with midface hypoplasia are not generally difficult to intubate, but may be difficult to ventilate.[2] An oral airway can be helpful in these patients. Identifying other vertebral or cardiac problems prior to anesthesia can be paramount. For example, patients with Klippel-Feil syndrome may have fusion of cervical vertebrae with limited neck flexion and/or extension. Patients with Down syndrome are at increased risk of atlantoaxial subluxation. In some of these cases, it may be crucial to limit extension of the neck during surgery, or it may be helpful to obtain plain films or computed tomography (CT) of the cervical spine before performing surgical procedures, to rule out cervical spine instability.

CRANIOFACIAL SYNOSTOSIS

Craniofacial synostosis refers to premature fusion of one or more of the cranial sutures and abnormal facial development. The most common syndromic craniofacial synostoses are Crouzon, Apert, and Pfeiffer syndromes. Patients usually have maxillary hypoplasia, poor growth of the midface, and a brachycephaly, or fusion of the coronal suture, which results in the appearance of a wide head (**Fig. 1**). In general, patients with Apert syndrome will have malformations of the hands and feet, such as syndactyly (baseball-glove appearance). Patients with Pfeiffer syndrome may have milder malformations of the digits, such as wide thumbs or toes. Among craniofacial patients, those with craniofacial synostosis may be the most likely to require a tracheostomy secondary to airway problems, approximately 48%.[1]

Apert Syndrome: Acrocephalosyndactyly

Background
Apert syndrome was first reported by Wheaton in 1894. However, it was Eugene Apert who expanded its description in 1906. This syndrome refers to the constellation of craniosynostosis, midfacial malformations, and symmetric syndactyly of the hands.[3] Although one of the most severe craniosynostoses, it is fortunately not a common entity. Apert syndrome has been reported in only 15 per 1 million live births.[4]

Apert syndrome is transmitted via autosomal dominant inheritance, although sporadic cases have also been reported. Increasing paternal age is associated with a higher incidence of Apert syndrome. An increased frequency of sperm mutations seems to be implicated.[5] Mutations in fibroblast growth factor receptor 2 (FGFR2)

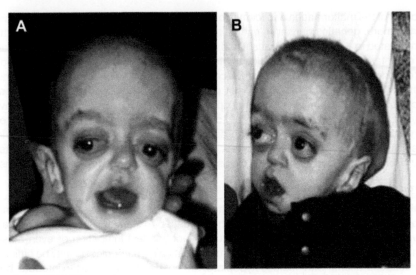

Fig. 1. (*A*, *B*) Pfeiffer syndrome.

on chromosome 10 are responsible for the autosomal dominant cases of this condition.[6]

Presentation

Apert syndrome can be diagnosed shortly after birth. Common facial features include orbital hypertelorism, proptosis, and down-slanting palpebral fissures. The midface is typically hypoplastic, which causes the mandible to appear protruded. A beaked nose, depressed nasal bridge, and deviated nasal septum are also observed.[3] The nasopharynx is small and the posterior choanae are narrowed.[3] All these features can cause significant nasal obstruction, leading to respiratory difficulty early in life. In addition, the small upper airway predisposes these patients to obstructive sleep apnea (OSA).

Oropharyngeal abnormalities are also commonly noted. A trapezoid-shaped mouth is characteristic. The palate is highly arched with lateral swellings and a median furrow.[3] Cleft soft palate or bifid uvula is found in approximately 75% cases.[7] Eustachian tube dysfunction is also common. Together, these two factors lead to frequent episodes of otitis media.

Hearing loss is frequently seen in patients with Apert syndrome. It is usually bilateral, and conductive hearing loss accounts for up to 80% of cases.[8] Middle ear effusion and a congenitally fixed stapes footplate are common causes of conductive hearing loss in this population. However, middle ear pathology is not the only contributor to hearing loss in these patients. Inner ear malformations, such as a dilated vestibule, malformed lateral semicircular canal, and cochlear dysplasia have also been reported.[8]

Workup

Although the diagnosis of Apert syndrome can be made clinically, a genetic test to detect mutations in FGFR2 is available. Skull and limb radiographs are helpful in detecting specific skeletal abnormalities. CT scanning with 3-dimensional reconstruction can be of paramount value in preoperative planning. In addition, a hearing evaluation is necessary in all patients with Apert syndrome. A flexible nasopharyngoscopy can be useful in assessing the anatomy of choanae and upper airway. Although the diagnosis of OSA can often be made by history and examination alone, polysomnography remains the gold standard.

Management

Positional changes and a nasopharyngeal or oropharyngeal airway may suffice in treating mild obstruction. Nasal secretions should be controlled with gentle suctioning and judicious use of nasal decongestants. Upper respiratory infections should be carefully managed, as they can exacerbate respiratory difficulties. It is also very important to effectively treat otitis media. Although acute infections can be effectively treated with oral antibiotics, chronic middle ear effusions are frequently treated with myringotomy and insertion of ventilation tubes.

In patients with OSA, continuous positive airway pressure may be used to keep the airway open.[9] Tonsillectomy and adenoidectomy may be necessary to help relieve OSA.

> HAZARD! If an adenoidectomy is necessary in patients with cleft palate, a conservative surgical approach should be used, given the risk of velopharyngeal insufficiency.

In severely affected children a tracheostomy may be necessary.

Craniofacial reconstruction is performed in a staged fashion. At around 9 to11 months, a cranio-orbital decompression is performed to increase the space in the anterior cranial vault and the orbit. The procedure entails osteotomies of the anterior cranial vault and upper orbits, and bicoronal suture release.[10] This procedure may need to be repeated if the child develops intracranial hypertension. A midline (facial bipartition) split combined with further reshaping of the cranial vault is performed later at age 5 to 7 years.[10] This procedure normalizes the arc of the midface, widens the maxillary arch, and shifts the orbits closer to the midline. The newly assembled midface is advanced horizontally to increase the orbital and zygomatic depth.[10] Le Fort I osteotomies with horizontal advancement must be performed to advance the maxilla and improve malocclusion.[10] A genioplasty may also be performed to help address the lower face deformity.[10]

Crouzon Syndrome: Craniofacial Dysostosis

Background

Crouzon syndrome is characterized by craniosynostosis, proptosis, shallow orbits, and maxillary hypoplasia.[3] This entity occurs in 15 to 16 per 1 million newborns.[11] The main form of inheritance is autosomal dominant with variable penetrance, although sporadic mutations also give rise to some cases. Increasing paternal age seems to play a role.[12] Similarly to Apert syndrome, mutations in FGFR2 are implicated in this syndrome, although the codons involved are different. Recently, a mutation in the transmembrane region of FGFR3 has been observed in these patients.[13]

Presentation

Patients with Crouzon syndrome are characterized by microcephaly, shallow orbits, and a long forehead.[14] The diagnosis may be clear at birth, or may manifest itself later during the first year of life.[3] Ocular proptosis, a feature seen in all the cases, occurs secondarily to the shallow orbits.[14] Cleft lip and palate do not occur frequently. Maxillary hypoplasia leads to a constricted dental arch, which causes the palate to appear high-arched.[3] A beaked nose and a deviated septum can occur, leading to nasal obstruction.[14] Atresia of the nasopharynx and hypopharynx can lead to respiratory distress.[15] The size of the maxillary sinus is significantly reduced.[16] Atresia of the external auditory canals occurs in 13% of cases.[3] Malalignment of the pinna has also been reported.[17] Otitis media and abnormalities of the ossicular chain can occur, and lead to conductive hearing loss.[17] These patients can also develop sensorineural and mixed hearing loss.[17]

Workup

Genetic testing for FGFR2 mutations is available. Most laboratories perform sequence analysis of select exons on the gene, but targeted mutation analysis can also be ordered. Prenatal testing is an option that may be valuable in identifying patients who may have difficulty breathing at birth.

Despite advances in imaging modalities, plain films of the skull remain useful in confirming the diagnosis. Three-dimensional CT scanning remains the best method for delineating the anatomic abnormalities and guiding surgical management.[18] As in patients with Apert syndrome, flexible nasopharyngoscopy can help assess the upper airway. Obstructive sleep apnea can ensue secondary to the midface abnormalities.[18] A polysomnogram is diagnostic. Given the high incidence of hearing loss in these patients, audiologic examination should be performed routinely.

Management

Because of the abnormal midface, nasopharynx, and hypopharynx, one of the main concerns becomes securing the airway from an early age. Some patients will require a tracheostomy shortly after birth. Because many patients undergo staged reconstruction, the tracheostomy may be left in place until all midface surgical procedures are completed.[18]

Similarly to Apert syndrome, multiple reconstructive procedures are necessary, with the first cranio-orbital decompression performed early in infancy at 9 to 11 months unless intracranial hypertension ensues.[10] Later in childhood, at approximately 7 to 9 years of age, the final cranial vault reconstruction is performed and the midface deformity is addressed with a facial bipartition or a Le Fort III osteotomy.[10] A separate Le Fort I osteotomy is needed to restore normal occlusion. This procedure is typically done during adolescence, at 13 to 15 years in females and 15 to 17 years in males.[10] Ancillary procedures such as a genioplasty are performed to address the mandibular deformity.[19]

Finally, because of the different otologic pathologies associated with this syndrome, close otologic and audiologic follow-up is recommended.[17]

CHARGE Association

Background

In 1979, Hall and Hittner reported the first cases of patients with CHARGE association in separate publications. Thus this association is also known as Hall-Hittner syndrome. In 1981, the acronym CHARGE was introduced by Pagon and colleagues. The letters stand for:

    Coloboma
    Heart defects
    Atresia choanae
    Retarded growth and development
    Genital hypoplasia
    Ear anomalies/deafness.

This association of anomalies has an incidence ranging from 0.1 to 1.2 per 10,000.[20] CHARGE is transmitted via an autosomal dominant pattern of inheritance. Mutations in the CHD7 gene, which codes for a DNA helicase, are present in more than 75% of cases.[20] The mutations are usually sporadic, although gonadal mosaicism and familial inheritance have been reported.[21]

Presentation

Patients with the classic 4Cs, namely (1) choanal atresia, (2) coloboma, (3) character-istic ears, and (4) cranial nerve anomalies, are very likely to have CHARGE syndrome.[20] Choanal atresia presents early and dramatically in life, with respiratory difficulty. Atresia may be membranous or bony, and bilateral or unilateral. In some cases, the presence of a cleft lip and palate can substitute for choanal atresia.[20] Patients with CHARGE have flat facies with sloping of the forehead and flattened tip of the nose. The ear is cup-shaped with a hypoplastic lobule, resulting from cartilage deficiency in the outer ear and lack of innervation from the facial nerve to the intrinsic ear muscles.[20] Asymmetric cranial nerve (CN) anomalies can be seen in these patients. Anosmia due to absence or dysfunction of the olfactory nerve (CN I), facial nerve palsy (CN VII), and sensorineural hearing loss (CN VIII) are observed.[20] Further-more, anomalies attributable to CN IX, X, and XI can lead to swallowing difficulties, esophageal reflux, and velopharyngeal insufficiency.[20] Hearing loss occurs frequently, and can be conductive or sensorineural. In addition to an abnormal CN VIII, patients may have a hypoplastic incus, Mondini defect (abnormal development of the cochlea resulting in less than 2.5 turns), or absent semicircular canal.[20]

Workup

Genetic testing is performed to confirm the diagnosis. Because of the classic middle and inner ear deformities associated with CHARGE, a CT of temporal bone is valuable. An audiogram and auditory brainstem response (ABR) are performed to assess the type and severity of hearing loss.[20] Imaging is very useful in delineating the shape of the choanae. Radiographic visualization of the olfactory tract and other CNs should also be performed.

Management

Bilateral choanal atresia can lead to an airway emergency. As always, stabilizing the airway should be a priority. Endotracheal intubation should be performed in the pres-ence of a pediatric anesthesiologist and/or otolaryngologist.[20] A tracheostomy may be needed in some cases. Surgical correction of choanal atresia can be challenging but should be attempted (**Fig. 2**). An endoscopic approach can be used first, and a trans-palatal approach used if the endoscopic surgery fails. When appropriate, hearing amplification should be started. Cochlear implants may be an option; however, the ear anatomy should be studied and presence of the eighth nerve should be confirmed by CT and/or magnetic resonance imaging (MRI).[22] Speech perception and language outcomes are difficult to assess in patients with developmental delay or other limitations.

PEARLS & PITFALLS: *Bilateral choanal atresia will often present as an airway emergency.*

CHROMOSOME-22 DELETION SYNDROMES/22q11.2 DELETION SYNDROMES

Various syndromes can occur as a result of chromosome-22 deletions, frequently a deletion of 22q11.2. The features can vary widely among the syndromes. The most frequently encountered in otolaryngology, DiGeorge, Velocardiofacial, and Opitz G/BBB syndromes, are described here in detail. In general, chromosome-22 deletion

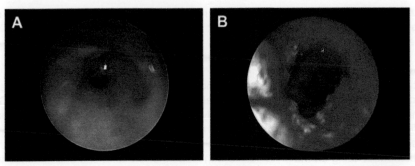

Fig. 2. (*A*) Choanal stenosis after initial repair. (*B*) Choanal stenosis intraoperatively after revision endoscopic repair.

syndromes can be remembered by the inappropriate mnemonic CATCH-22, which includes cardiac defects, abnormal facies, thymic aplasia or hypoplasia, cleft palate, and hypocalcemia. DiGeorge syndrome embodies this most closely. Many patients will have some developmental delay or learning difficulties. In addition, these patients may have laryngeal pathology, such as clefts or webs.

DiGeorge Syndrome

Background
DiGeorge syndrome is named after Dr Angelo DiGeorge, who in 1965 described an entity characterized by congenital absence of the parathyroid glands and thymus, which lead to hypocalcemia and immune deficiency, respectively. The deletion of chromosome 22q11.2, which encompasses more than 35 genes, is responsible for the abnormalities. Defective migration of the neural crest cells causes abnormal development of the third and fourth branchial pouches. As a consequence, structures derived from these pouches are affected.

This entity has been estimated to occur in 1 in 3000 to 6000 births.[23] De novo mutations are responsible for the deletion, although the syndrome can be inherited in an autosomal dominant fashion.[24] Males and females are equally affected, and there is no ethnic preference.[22]

Presentation
There is a high degree of phenotypical expression among patients affected with DiGeorge syndrome. Micrognathia is present and becomes subtle as the patient ages. The eyes appear hooded, and the nose has a broad root and a bulbous tip.[22] The palate is affected in the vast majority of those diagnosed with DiGeorge syndrome.[22] Overt and submucous cleft palate may occur, but cleft lip is uncommon.[25] The main functional issue is velopharyngeal weakness, which leads to hypernasal speech and nasal reflux. Laryngeal webs and vocal cord paralysis may also cause abnormal phonation.[22] All of these factors can contribute to speech delay. The average patient will begin speaking at 30 months.[22] Conductive hearing loss is present in approximately 45% of patients, and 10% have sensorineural loss. In general, patients have posteriorly rotated ears or a simple helix, but microtia and anotia can also occur.[22] Feeding difficulties, resulting from palatal clefting and/or swallowing problems, are common and can be distressing to parents.

Workup
The typical deletion is submicroscopic, and fluorescence in situ hybridization (FISH) has been the method of choice used to detect it. Atypical deletions cannot be

identified by this method. The polymerase chain reaction and the use of single-nucleotide polymorphism arrays are alternatives to FISH.[22] An audiology examination should be performed at an early age. Flexible nasopharyngoscopy is key in diagnosing submucous clefts, velopharyngeal insufficiency, and nasopharyngeal depth. Video-fluoroscopy during speech can be helpful as well. Because of the risk of malposition of the carotid arteries, imaging is necessary before performing a tonsillectomy[22] or other pharyngeal surgery, such as a pharyngoplasty for velopharyngeal insufficiency. A standard CT or MRI of the neck is sufficient. Magnetic resonance angiography or conventional angiography will demonstrate the position of the arteries as well. A CT (or MRI) of the temporal bone may be needed to assess for cochleovestibular malformations, depending on the patient's hearing loss.

PEARLS & PITFALLS: *Preoperative imaging is recommended in children with c chromosome 22 deletion syndrome undergoing pharyngeal surgery because of the risk of malposition of the carotid arteries.*

Management
Hearing problems should be treated appropriately, with surgery and/or assistive hearing devices as indicated by the patient's type of hearing loss. Close attention should be paid to speech development, and referral to a speech pathologist should be made when adequate. Correction of the palatal defect should be undertaken if the patient is an adequate candidate. In cases of hypodynamic velopharynx, hypernasality may persist after surgery.[22] Adenoidectomy is not routinely performed because the adenoid aids in nasopharyngeal closure. Ventilation tubes should be placed if the patient is affected by otitis media. Gastroesophageal reflux, if present, should be treated,[23] especially if it is contributing to feeding difficulties or failure to thrive.

Velocardiofacial Syndrome

Background
First described in 1978, velocardiofacial syndrome (VCFS) is characterized by cleft palate and hypernasal speech, cardiac abnormalities, learning disability, and specific facial features.[26] This entity is also caused by a deletion of 22q11.2.[27] It can be transmitted in an autosomal dominant fashion, but most cases occur as a result of de novo deletions or translocations.[25] Some patients do not have a detectable deletion but still carry the diagnosis based on clinical features. Phenotypical variability is common, and the patient may appear normal. Thus, a high degree of suspicion is needed. The prevalence of VCFS in the United States is 1 in 2000.[28]

Presentation
VCFS is the most common syndrome associated with clefting of the secondary palate. Approximately 98% cases have a palatal cleft.[26] Other features include pharyngeal hypotonia and hypernasal speech.[25]

HAZARD! *Velopharyngeal insufficiency can result from these anomalies as well as small adenoid size, pharyngeal musculature hypotonia, and platybasia (obtuse angulation of the cranial base).*[23]

Because of the shape of the skull base, the maxilla appears long and the malar eminence is flattened. The mandible appears retrognathic and the nasal root is broad. These features may mimic the classic adenoid facies.[25] Narrow palpebral fissures and hypertelorism are additional findings.[25] Small and cupped ears, thickened helices, and abnormally positioned auricles can also be seen.[25] Up to 90% of children can have chronic otitis media with associated conductive hearing loss.[25] It has been postulated that the high incidence of middle ear disease results from anatomic abnormalities, palatal clefting, and Eustachian tube dysfunction.[25] Hearing loss can also occur secondary to narrowing of the external auditory canals and ossicular abnormalities. A sensorineural cause can be a contributing factor.[25] Vocal fold nodules as a result of laryngeal hyperfunction can be seen, and are thought to arise from compensatory speech mechanisms.[25]

Workup

VCFS is usually diagnosed by physical examination. The diagnosis can be confirmed by FISH analysis with great accuracy.[27] When a submucous cleft palate is suspected, palpation during oral examination can be helpful. Nasopharyngoscopy allows for examination of the nasal surface of the velum. The musculus uvulae may be absent or hypoplastic in patients with occult submucous cleft palate.[25] In addition, nasopharyngoscopy can aid in diagnosing medial displacement of the carotid arteries.[25] Endoscopy to the level of the larynx allows for examination of the glottis, as vocal fold nodules are common incidental findings. Magnetic resonance angiography is an option for all patients before undergoing surgical correction of velopharyngeal insufficiency,[29] but a CT of the neck may provide enough information. An audiogram should be performed, given the high rate of middle ear infections.

> PEARLS & PITFALLS: *It is recommended that all patients diagnosed with anterior glottic webs undergo FISH testing because of the strong association with chromosome 22q microdeletion.[30]*

Management

Adenoidectomy should not routinely be performed in these patients. If it is absolutely necessary, some investigators suggest a selective superior adenoidectomy.[25] Early myringotomy and placement of ventilating tubes is recommended to avoid permanent complications from chronic otitis media.[25] Cleft palate should be repaired to improve speech and feeding. However, speech disorders do not usually resolve with isolated palate repair. Further reconstructive procedures, such as pharyngeal flap surgery, are commonly needed.[27] Pharyngoplasty may be needed for patients with hyponasal speech without a cleft palate.

Opitz G/BBB Syndrome

Background

In 1969 Opitz and Frias described a constellation of findings in the "G Family," hence the syndrome was known as the Opitz-Frias syndrome or G syndrome.[31] Opitz, Summitt, and Smith described a similar syndrome in 3 other families with the initial B,[32] hence the BBB syndrome. Opitz G/BBB syndrome involves midline defects including distinct facial features as well as cleft lip, palate, laryngeal cleft, and hypospadias. Opitz G/BBB syndrome is most often X-linked, but can be autosomal dominant. This syndrome affects 1 in 50,000 to 100,000 males.[33] The autosomal dominant form has been linked to chromosome-22 deletions as in patients with DiGeorge syndrome or velocardiofacial syndrome.[34,35]

Presentation

Patients' distinct facial features include hypertelorism, anteverted nares, prominent forehead, narrow palpebral fissures with epicanthal folds, and widow's peak.[33,36] Many patients will also have genitourinary abnormalities, such as hypospadias or cryptorchidism. About 50% of patients with the syndrome will have a cleft lip and/or palate. One of the unique otolaryngologic features is a laryngeal cleft. Laryngeal cleft occurs in approximately 30% of patients with Opitz-Frias G/BBB syndrome.[36] The grade or type of cleft may vary as well as severity of presenting symptoms. Symptoms of a laryngeal cleft may include cough, stridor, dysphagia, or other signs of aspiration. Other malformations such as congenital heart defections, imperforate anus, or midline brain defects occur in fewer than 50% of patients.

Workup

Genetic testing should be performed for the MID1 (midline-1) gene, but the diagnosis is made clinically. Genetic testing will identify mutations in 15% to 45% of patients with the syndrome.[2] Patients should have a thorough physical examination, echocardiogram, and evaluation of speech pathology with video swallow study. In cases of severe respiratory distress and more subtle symptoms, such as cough or chronic aspiration, it is important to perform a direct laryngoscopy and spread the arytenoids to evaluate for the presence of a laryngeal cleft.[37]

Management

As with any craniofacial anomaly, ensuring a safe airway is most important for these patients. In cases of respiratory distress, a tracheotomy may be needed. When aspiration is diagnosed, it should be treated with proton-pump inhibitors or histamine-2 blockers. If a laryngeal cleft is present, it merits repair. An endoscopic approach can be considered in patients with a grade I or II laryngeal cleft (**Fig. 3**).[38] Open laryngofissure and repair are often required in patients with larger clefts.[39] Sometimes surgical repair of the cleft is delayed and a temporary feeding tube may be needed. Cleft lip and palate are treated in a standard fashion.

CONGENITAL NASAL PYRIFORM APERTURE STENOSIS
Background

Congenital nasal pyriform aperture stenosis (CNPAS) (**Fig. 4**) was first described by Brown and colleagues in 1989. This condition can occur in an isolated fashion or be associated with other anomalies such as holoprosencephaly, hypopituitarism, and a single central megaincisor.[40] The degree of stenosis is variable, thus making the true incidence of the condition difficult to ascertain.[41] CNPAS typically occurs bilaterally, and can be commonly misdiagnosed as choanal stenosis or atresia. The abnormalities in development leading to this condition are not clearly understood. Abnormalities of chromosomes 7, 13, or 18 have been reported.[39]

Presentation

One of the first presenting symptoms in patients with CNPAS is nasal obstruction with cyclic cyanosis relieved by crying.[40] Difficulty breathing during feeding is also observed.[39] It is difficult to pass a catheter through the anterior nares. Anterior

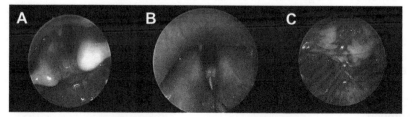

Fig. 3. (A) Grade I laryngeal cleft, which can be subtle on initial laryngoscopy. (B) Probe between arytenoids demonstrates cleft down to level of the vocal folds. (C) Sutures in place at posterior arytenoids are after endoscopic repair of the cleft.

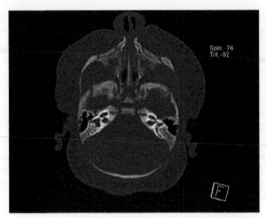

Spin -76
Tilt -92

Fig. 4. Computed tomography demonstrates nasal pyriform aperture stenosis.

rhinoscopy is difficult because of the small nasal fossa and submucous bone protrusion.[42] Severe obstruction leads to increased work of breathing, which in turn may cause failure to thrive.

Workup

History and clinical examination are usually sufficient to make the correct diagnosis. Flexible laryngoscopy is usually performed. However, a CT scan should always be performed to confirm the clinical suspicion. The study of choice is a fine-cut CT without contrast from the palate to the orbit.[40] The confirmatory finding is overgrowth of the nasal process with narrowing of the nasal passages.[40] Three-dimensional CT is helpful in preoperative planning.[43] Imaging will also confirm or rule out the presence of other midline abnormalities. MRI should be performed in patients with a central megaincisor, given the association with holoprosencephaly and pituitary insufficiency.

Management

The first step in managing these patients should always be securing the airway. Some patients may not need any intervention other than careful observation. An oral airway or McGovern nipple may be sufficient initially.[40] If the obstructive symptoms are mild, conservative management with careful use of nasal decongestants or even saline drops may be attempted. The nasal airway may improve as the patient ages, usually by age 6 months.[44] If the obstruction is severe enough to cause respiratory distress, endotracheal intubation should be performed. Surgical management is indicated in those patients with severe respiratory compromise, failure to thrive, or nonresponsiveness to medical management.[40] A sublabial surgical approach can be used to widen the floor of the nose bilaterally with an otologic drill. Inferior turbinate reduction may be adjunctively performed.[40] Keeping nasal stents in place postoperatively helps maintain airway patency. There is a risk of restenosis postoperatively, particularly if meticulous irrigation is not performed. An endoscopic technique has been attempted by some, but may not provide adequate visualization in infants.[45]

MOEBIUS SYNDROME
Background

Moebius syndrome is named after Paul Moebius, a German neurologist, who in 1888 compared his cases of paralysis of CN VI and VII with other similar reports.[46,47]

However, the first description of Moebius syndrome dates back to 1880 when von Graefe discussed a combination of congenital bilateral CN VI and CN VII palsy.[48] Since then, the definition has been expanded to include other cranial nerve abnormalities. From most frequent to least frequent, these include XII, X, IX, III, VIII, V, IV, and XI.[49] In addition, this entity is also associated with chest wall defects, mental retardation, and limb malformations,[50] particularly club foot. The etiology remains unknown, but a disruption in the embryologic development of the subclavian artery seems to play a role.[38] Exposure to misoprostol and thalidomide in utero is strongly correlated with Moebius syndrome.[49] Almost all cases are sporadic, but some autosomal dominant and recessive cases have been reported.[49] Moebius syndrome is very rare, and the prevalence has been reported as low as 0.002%.[51]

Presentation

Early in infancy, patients experience difficulty sucking, drooling and incomplete eye closure.[49] The face is motionless, leading to the classic "masklike" facies. Bilateral horizontal gaze palsy is also classically found. Mandibular micrognathia and retrognathia, microglossia, and a fissure tongue are common characteristics.[49] In addition, a high-arched palate, bifid uvula or cleft palate may be seen.[49] Secondary to palatal abnormalities, recurrent otitis media and velopharyngeal incompetence ensue.[49] Thus hearing loss, either from chronic otitis media or palsy of the eighth nerve, occurs frequently. Articulation is very limited secondary to glossal and facial paralysis. Bilateral vocal cord paralysis, although rare, has been reported.[52] Hence, airway obstruction and inability to protect the airway leading to aspiration are potential life-threatening complications.

Workup

When the diagnosis of Moebius syndrome is suspected, patients should undergo CT or MRI scanning to rule out brain lesions that could be responsible or contribute to the CN abnormalities.[53] Careful audiologic examination and auditory brainstem response (ABR) testing should be performed to evaluate hearing and brainstem deficits.[52] In addition, patients should undergo ophthalmology evaluation to assess for visual defects.[52] A flexible nasopharyngoscopy is helpful in evaluating velopharyngeal competence and vocal cord mobility.

Management

The early management of these patients is mainly supportive. In the case of airway obstruction, a tracheostomy may be required. Nutritional support via a gastrostomy tube may be necessary. A speech pathologist should be consulted to improve oropharyngeal coordination and aid in swallowing and speech development. A hearing evaluation should be performed. Tympanostomy tubes may be necessary in patients with chronic otitis media. Because of the inability to close the eye, it is imperative to use artificial lubrication and tape the eye closed during sleep to prevent corneal ulceration and conjunctivitis.

> PEARLS & PITFALLS: *Eye precautions must be remembered in the management of Moebius syndrome.*

Tendon slings, temporalis muscle transfer, and gold weights can be used to aid with eye closure.[49] Lack of facial expression causes significant distress to patients because it impairs social interaction. At present, the procedure of choice performed to provide facial reanimation is a neurovascular free muscle transfer.[49] The pectoralis minor and gracilis muscles are commonly used. The motor branch to the masseter, partial hypoglossal, or accessory nerve can be successfully grafted to produce a smile.[49]

MANDIBULOFACIAL DYSOSTOSIS

Mandibulofacial dysostosis syndromes include Treacher-Collins syndrome and Nager syndrome. Patients with Nager acrofacial dysostosis have mandibulofacial dysostosis and malformed upper limbs, and can have similar airway problems to patients with Treacher-Collins syndrome.[54]

Treacher-Collins Syndrome

Background

Treacher-Collins syndrome is relatively common among the craniofacial syndromes, and can occur along a phenotypically wide spectrum of mild to severe, even within families. The syndrome is autosomal dominant but can also occur de novo. It occurs in approximately 1 in 50,000 live births. Mutations in the TCOF1 gene lead to low amounts of the treacle protein, which reduces the number of cranial neural crest cells migrating to the first and second pharyngeal arches.[55]

Presentation

Because phenotype may vary, presentation varies significantly. Mildly affected patients may not present with any problems, whereas severely affected patients may present at birth with dyspnea or apnea as a result of micrognathia. In general, patients with Treacher-Collins syndrome have easily recognizable facial features, including down-slanting palpebral fissures, malar and maxillary hypoplasia, and microtia/atresia. Malocclusion can also be seen. These features may be present in one parent. Auricular abnormalities and hearing loss are common. Some children can present with a failed newborn hearing screening test. Most investigators approximate that hearing loss occurs in 50% of patients with Treacher-Collins syndrome.[56] Of 30 patients in one practice, 37% of patients had cleft palate, all had hearing loss (93% conductive, 7% mixed), and 77% had hypernasal and/or hyponasal speech.[57]

Workup

Genetic testing for Treacher-Collins syndrome, specifically TCOF1, confirms the diagnosis. Patients with airway problems should be evaluated by laryngoscopy. Given the high incidence of hearing loss, all patients should have a thorough audiology evaluation. Patients will likely need a CT of the temporal bone to evaluate development of the ossicles and evaluate for other causes of congenital hearing loss. An MRI may be indicated for evaluation of the internal auditory canal. Additional imaging is typically necessary for preoperative planning. A craniofacial CT scan should be ordered before mandibular distraction.

Management

Management of airway and feeding problems is most important in infants. Most patients can be managed conservatively. For feeding problems and possible aspiration, early evaluation with a speech pathologist is important. For airway problems, some patients may be candidates for mandibular distraction, successfully avoiding tracheotomy, or as a means to decannulation.[58] In one large craniofacial practice, 41% of 59 patients with mandibulofacial dysostosis required a tracheostomy.[1] Four of 50 (8%) patients with Treacher-Collins syndrome in another group required a tracheostomy, 1 of whom died and 3 of whom had mandibular distraction; 23% had a cleft palate repair.[59] In general, the cleft palate can be repaired at about age 9 to 12 months. Hearing loss is usually treated initially with hearing aids. Orthognathic surgery is usually performed between 13 and 18 years of age. Reconstruction of the cheek or maxilla can be performed as well, including eyelid correction, zygoma, and lateral orbit reconstruction. In a group of 50 patients in Poland, an average of 5.2 operations, from orthognathic surgery to auricular reconstruction, were performed per patient.[60]

Congenital bilateral conductive hearing loss is most commonly treated with a bone-anchored conduction hearing aid with a soft headband for children younger than 3 or 4 years. When old enough for surgery, a bone-anchored system is a good option,[61] including the Baha for Treacher-Collins patients.[62] A pinna epithesis can be used in combination with a Baha.[56] Alternatively, the auricle can be reconstructed, usually at between 8 and 10 years old. Middle ear surgery can be performed but has shown mixed results.[63] Implantable hearing aids may also be an option.[64]

OCULOAURICULAR-VERTEBRAL SPECTRUM

The syndromes of the oculoauricular-vertebral spectrum (OAVS) refer to anomalies of the eyes, ears, and vertebral column. Affected patients may have mild to severe forms along the spectrum. Similarly to Treacher-Collins syndrome, this category of anomalies tends to affect the first and second branchial arches. This entity includes hemifacial microsomia and Goldenhar syndrome. Hemifacial microsomia is now called craniofacial microsomia to better encompass the full process of the disease, which includes poor growth of the cranium, facial skeleton, and soft tissues of the face. The most notable growth asymmetry occurs in the mandible. Growth of the maxilla may be restricted as well. As a result, sleep-disordered breathing is common.[65] Vertebral and eye problems are rare, but hearing problems can be common, likely a result of abnormalities of the ossicles, auricle, or external auditory canal. OAVS likely occurs in about 1 in 20,000 births.[55] Some OAVS can be associated with a constellation of anomalies known as VACTERL.[66] Patients with different syndromes can have these VACTERL signs: Vertebral anomalies, Anal atresia, Cardiovascular malformations, Tracheoesophageal fistula, Esophageal atresia, Renal anomalies, and Limb defects. For the otolaryngologist, it is especially important to keep in mind the possibility of tracheoesophageal fistula as a cause for feeding difficulties or respiratory distress.

Goldenhar Syndrome

Background
Goldenhar syndrome consists of a classic triad of craniofacial microsomia, ocular dermoid cysts, and vertebral anomalies. Most cases are sporadic. However, autosomal recessive and autosomal dominant familial cases have been reported.[67] There are reports of an associated with chromosome 22q11.2 deletion,[68] as well as other genes. The etiology is most likely multifactorial.[69] Reduced blood flow to the soft tissues during development is one possible explanation.

Presentation
Facial asymmetry can include craniofacial microsomia and malocclusion, typically with macrostomia or lateral cleft of the lip. Ear malformations can occur as anotia, microtia, or preauricular tags. Otolaryngologists, especially preoperatively, should be aware of congenital facial nerve weakness and abnormal facial nerve anatomy in patients with microtia. Preauricular tags or other similar soft-tissue deformities can occur anywhere from the tragus to the oral commissure. Eye malformations may include anophthalmia, microphthalmia, epibulbar dermoids, and eyelid colobomas. Cleft lip and/or palate, and renal and gastrointestinal abnormalities can be observed.[70]

Vertebral anomalies can include a wide range of problems at all levels within the spine.[71]

Workup

Genetic workup often does not show any chromosomal abnormalities. Similar to Treacher-Collins syndrome, patients with Goldenhar syndrome will require audiograms and temporal bone imaging. A craniofacial CT is necessary to evaluate the temporomandibular joint. Radiographs of the spine may be necessary as well.

Management

Management of patients with OAVS depends on the specific phenotype. These patients are less likely to have a tracheotomy than patients with other syndromes causing craniofacial microsomia or micrognathia. Approximately 22% will require tracheostomy.[1] Macrostomia repair can be performed as early as age 2 to 3 months. Minor preauricular deformities can be surgically corrected as well. However, definitive reconstruction of the ear is delayed until the patient is about 5 years old, as with other patients with microtia. Hearing loss is managed based on the patient's type and severity of loss. Orbital dystopia may be corrected in severely affected children, with cranial remodeling between ages 8 and 12 months. Distraction osteogenesis may be performed in infancy for airway compromise and/or later during the teenage years for correction of malocclusion and cosmesis. The type and timing of the surgical repair may vary, depending on the type of mandibular deformity.

STICKLER SYNDROME
Background

Stickler syndrome is a subtype of collagenopathy, specifically types II and XI. Gunnar B. Stickler first described the syndrome in 1965. This condition is thought to be dominantly inherited, although there is likely no single genetic entity that causes Stickler syndrome.[72] The phenotype of patients with Stickler syndrome may vary significantly, making the diagnosis and identification of criteria for diagnosis difficult. Mutations in the COL11A2 gene can cause autosomal dominant nonocular Stickler syndrome.[73] Various other COL genes have been linked to autosomal recessive Stickler syndrome.

Presentation

Many patients with Stickler syndrome will have Pierre Robin sequence, a retrognathic mandible thought to lead to elevation of the tongue and incomplete closure of the palatine shelves. In addition to retrognathia and cleft palate, these patients present with other symptoms of connective tissue disease, including skeletal abnormality such as osteoarthritis, maxillary hypoplasia, and ocular anomalies. Ocular abnormalities in Stickler syndrome may include retinal detachment, glaucoma, premature cataracts, high myopia, optically empty vitreous cavities, and retinal pigmentary changes.[74] Patients often have a progressive sensorineural hearing loss.[75]

Workup

Genetic workup is valuable in any patient with craniofacial abnormalities. Patients with Robin sequence should have an ophthalmology consultation because of the association between Stickler syndrome and vision loss. A speech pathology consultation is recommended to evaluate feeding. As with all craniofacial patients, an audiogram should be performed regularly. Evaluation of the airway by flexible and/or rigid laryngoscopy may be necessary. A maxillofacial CT scan may be helpful in delineating upper airway anatomy.

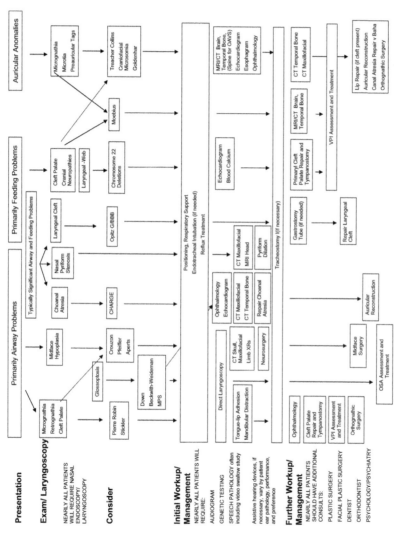

Fig. 5. Summary of management of patients with craniofacial syndromes. CT, computed tomography; MPS, mucopolysaccharidosis; MRI, magnetic resonance imaging; OAVS, oculoauricular-vertebral spectrum; OSA, obstructive sleep apnea; VPI, velopharyngeal insufficiency; XRs, radiography.

Management

For infants, managing airway and feeding problems is most important. Airway intervention may include positioning, tongue-lip adhesion, distraction osteogenesis, or tracheotomy. Feeding problems may require a feeding tube. Because most patients will have chronic otitis media as a result of the cleft palate, ear tubes may be placed at the time of the cleft palate repair, if not earlier. Cleft palate is repaired at around age 9 months. Amplification with hearing aids is recommended for sensorineural hearing loss. If distraction was not performed early in life, it may be necessary in late childhood or early adolescence if malocclusion persists.

ALGORITHM

The algorithm shown in **Fig. 5** summarizes the management of patients with craniofacial syndromes.

REFERENCES

1. Sculerati N, Gottlieb MD, Zimbler MS, et al. Airway management in children with major craniofacial anomalies. Laryngoscope 1998;108(12):1806–12.
2. Nargozian C. The airway in patients with craniofacial abnormalities. Paediatr Anaesth 2004;14:53–9.
3. Gorlin RJ, Cohen MM Jr, Hennekam RC. Syndromes with craniosynostosis: general aspects and well-known syndromes. In: Syndromes of the head and neck. 4th edition. New York: Oxford University Press; 2001. p. 654–70.
4. Cohen MM Jr, Kreiborg S. New indirect method for estimating the birth prevalence of the Apert's syndrome. Int J Oral Maxillofac Surg 1992;21:107–9.
5. Glaser RL, Broman KW, Schulman RL, et al. The paternal-age effect in Apert syndrome is due, in part, to the increased frequency of mutations in sperm. Am J Hum Genet 2003;73(4):939–47.
6. Chen L, Li D, Li C, et al. A Ser250trp substitution in mouse fibroblast growth factor receptor 2 (FGFR2) results in craniosynostosis. Bone 2003;33:169–78.
7. Kreiborg S, Cohen MM Jr. The oral manifestations of Apert syndrome. J Craniofac Genet Dev Biol 1992;2(1):41–8.
8. Zhou G, Schwartz LT, Gopen Q. Inner ear anomalies and conductive hearing loss in children with Apert syndrome: an overlooked otologic aspect. Otol Neurotol 2009;30(2):184–9.
9. Chen H. Apert syndrome. In: Allanson JE, editor. Atlas of genetic diagnosis and counseling. Totowa (NJ): Humana Press Inc.; 2006. p. 61–9.
10. Posnick JC, Ruiz RL. The craniofacial dysostosis syndromes: current surgical thinking and future directions. Cleft Palate Craniofac J 2000;37(5):433.
11. Cohen MM Jr, Kreiborg S. Birth prevalence studies of the Crouzon syndrome: comparison of direct and indirect methods. Clin Genet 1992;41(1):12–5.
12. Glaser RL, Jiang W, Boyadjiev SA, et al. Paternal origin of FGFR2 mutations in sporadic cases of Crouzon syndrome and Pfeiffer syndrome. Am J Hum Genet 2000;66(3):768–77.
13. Wilkes D, Rutland P, Pulleyn LJ, et al. A recurrent mutation, ala391glu, in the transmembrane region of FGFR3 causes Crouzon syndrome and acanthosis nigricans. J Med Genet 1996;33(9):744–8.
14. Gilbert P. Crouzon's syndrome. In: A-Z of syndromes and inherited disorders. 3rd edition. Great Britain: Ashford Colour Press Ltd; 2000. p. 76–8.

15. Katzen JT, McCarthy JG. Syndromes involving craniosynostosis and midface hypoplasia. Otolaryngol Clin North Am 2000;33(6):1257–84.
16. Song SY, Hong JW, Roh TS, et al. Volume and distances of the maxillary sinus in craniofacial deformities with midfacial hypoplasia. Otolaryngol Head Neck Surg 2009;141(5):614–20.
17. Orvidas LJ, Fabry LB, Diacova S, et al. Hearing and otopathology in Crouzon syndrome. Laryngoscope 1999;109(9):1372–5.
18. Goodrich JT. Craniofacial syndromes. In: Albright AL, Adelson PD, Pollack IF, editors. Principles and practice of pediatric neurosurgery. 2nd edition. New York: Thieme Medical Publishers Inc; 2008. p. 289–309.
19. Posnick JC. Crouzon syndrome: basic dysmorphology and staging of reconstruction. In: Greenberg AM, Prein J, editors. Craniomaxillofacial reconstructive and corrective bone surgery: principles of internal fixation using the AO/ASIF technique. New York: Springer-Verlag New York Inc; 2002. p. 713–26.
20. Blake KD, Prasad C. CHARGE Syndrome. Orphanet J Rare Dis 2006;1:34.
21. Jongmans MC, Hoefsloot LH, van der Donk KP, et al. Familial CHARGE syndrome and the CHD7 gene: a recurrent missense mutation, intrafamilial recurrence and variability. Am J Med Genet A 2008;146(1):43–50.
22. Arndt S, Laszig R, Beck R, et al. Spectrum of hearing disorders and their management in children with CHARGE syndrome. Otol Neurotol 2010;31(1): 67–73.
23. McDonald-McGinn DM, Sullivan KE. Chromosome 22q11.2 deletion syndrome (DiGeorge syndrome/velocardiofacial syndrome). Medicine (Baltimore) 2011; 90(1):1–18.
24. Kobrynski LJ, Sullivan KE. Velocardiofacial syndrome, DiGeorge syndrome: the chromosome 22q11.2 deletion syndromes. Lancet 2007;370(9596):1443–52.
25. McDonald-McGinn DM, Kirschner R, Goldmuntz E, et al. The Philadelphia story: the 22q11.2 deletion: report on 250 patients. Genet Couns 1999;10(1):11–24.
26. Ford LC, Sulprizio SL, Rasgon BM. Otolaryngological manifestations of velocardiofacial syndrome: a retrospective review of 35 patients. Laryngoscope 2000; 110(3 Pt 1):362–7.
27. Goldberg R, Motzkin B, Marion R, et al. Velo-cardiofacial syndrome: a review of 120 patients. Am J Med Genet 1993;45(3):313–9. Review.
28. Shprintzen RJ. Velo-cardio-facial syndrome: 30 years of study. Dev Disabil Res Rev 2008;14(1):3–10.
29. Mitnick RJ, Bello JA, Golding-Kushner KJ, et al. The use of magnetic resonance angiography prior to pharyngeal flap surgery in patients with velocardiofacial syndrome. Plast Reconstr Surg 1996;97(5):908–19.
30. Miyamoto RC, Cotton RT, Rope AF, et al. Association of anterior glottic webs with velocardiofacial syndrome (chromosome 22q11.2 deletion). Otolaryngol Head Neck Surg 2004;140(4):415–7.
31. Allanson JE. G syndrome: an unusual family. Am J Med Genet 1988;31(3): 637–42.
32. Opitz JM, Summitt RL, Smith DW. The BBB syndrome familial telecanthus with associated congenital anomalies. Birth Defects Orig Artic Ser (V) 1969;2:86–94.
33. Meroni G. X-Linked Opitz G/BBB Syndrome. In: Pagon RA, Bird TD, Dolan CR, et al, editors. Gene reviews [internet]. Seattle (WA): University of Washington; 1993–2004 [updated 2007 Jun 20].
34. Erickson RP, Diza de Stahl T, Bruder CE, et al. A patient with 22q11.2 deletion and Opitz syndrome-like phenotype has the same deletion as velocardiofacial patients. Am J Med Genet A 2007;143(24):3302–8.

35. Mcdonald-McGinn DM, Emanuel BS, Zackai EH. Autosomal dominant "Opitz" GBBB syndrome due to a 22q11.2 deletion. Am J Med Genet 1996;64(3):525–6.
36. Bershof JF, Guyuron B, Olsen MM. G syndrome: a review of the literature and a case report. J Craniomaxillofac Surg 1992;20(1):24–7.
37. Neubauer PD, Swibel Rosenthal LH, Wooten W, et al. Diagnosis of laryngeal cleft. American Academy of Otolaryngology Annual Meeting. San Francisco (CA); September 2011.
38. Rahbar R, Chen JL, Rosen RL, et al. Endoscopic repair of laryngeal cleft type I and type II: when and why? Laryngoscope 2009;119(9):1797–802.
39. Rahbar R, Rouillon I, Roger G, et al. The presentation and management of laryngeal cleft: a 10-year experience. Arch Otolaryngol Head Neck Surg 2006; 132(12):1335–41.
40. Robson CD, Hudgins PA. Pediatric airway disease. In: Som PM, Curtin HD, editors. Head and neck imaging. 4th edition. St Louis (MO): Mosby; 2003. p. 1521–93.
41. Tate JR, Sykes J. Congenital nasal pyriform aperture stenosis. Otolaryngol Clin North Am 2009;42(3):521–5.
42. Goldenberg D, Flax-Goldenberg R, Joachimn HZ, et al. Quiz case 1 (radiology forum). Arch Otolaryngol Head Neck Surg 2000;126(1):94–7.
43. Lee K, Yang C, Huang J, et al. Congenital pyriform aperture stenosis: surgery and evaluation with three dimensional computed tomography. Laryngoscope 2002; 112(5):918–21.
44. Lee J, Bent J, Ward R. Congenital nasal pyriform aperture stenosis: non-surgical management and long-term analysis. Int J Pediatr Otorhinolaryngol 2001;60(2): 167–72.
45. Brown O, Myer C, Manning S. Congenital nasal pyriform aperture stenosis. Laryngoscope 1989;99(1):86–91.
46. Möbius PJ. Uber angeborene doppelseitige Abducens-Facialis lahmung. Muench Med Wochenschr 1888;35:91–108 [in German].
47. Möbius PJ. Uber infantilen Kernschwund. Muench Med Wochenschr 1892;39: 17–58 [in German].
48. Von Graefe A. Diagnostik der Augenmuskellähmungen and Aetiologie und Pathogenese der Augenmuskellähmungen. In: Von Graefe A, Saemisch T, editors. Handbuch der Gesamten Augenheilkunde. (Handbook of Ophthalmology), vol. 6. Leipzig (Germany): W Engelmann; 1880. p. 60–7 [in German].
49. Carr MM, Ross DA, Zuker RM. Cranial nerve defects in congenital facial palsy. J Otolaryngol 1997;26:80–7.
50. Singham J, Manktelow R, Zuker RM. Möbius syndrome. Semin Plast Surg 2004; 18(1):39–46.
51. Verzijl HT, van der Zwaag B, Cruysberg JR, et al. Möbius syndrome redefined: a syndrome of rhombencephalic maldevelopment. Neurology 2003;61(3): 327–33.
52. Kanemoto N, Kanemoto K, Kamoda T, et al. A case of Moebius syndrome presenting with congenital bilateral vocal cord paralysis. Eur J Pediatr 2007; 166(8):831–3.
53. Gillberg C. Clinical child neuropsychiatry. Cambridge (United Kingdom): Cambridge University Press; 2003. p 229–30.
54. Friedman RA, Wood E, Pransky SM, et al. Nager acrofacial dysostosis: management of a difficult airway. Int J Pediatr Otorhinolaryngol 1996;35(1):69–72.
55. Passos-Bueno MR, Ornelas CC, Fanganiello RD. Syndromes of the first and second pharyngeal arches: a review. Am J Med Genet A 2009;149:1853–9.

56. Marres HA. Hearing loss in the Treacher-Collins syndrome. Adv Otorhinolaryngol 2002;61:209–15.
57. Vallino-Napoli LD. A profile of the features and speech in patients with mandibulofacial dysostosis. Cleft Palate Craniofac J 2002;39(6):623–34.
58. Miloro M. Mandibular distraction osteogenesis for pediatric airway management. J Oral Maxillofac Surg 2010;68(7):1512–23.
59. Thompson JT, Anderson PJ, David DJ. Treacher Collins syndrome: protocol management from birth to maturity. J Craniofac Surg 2009;20(6):2028–35.
60. Kobus K, Wojcicki P. Surgical treatment of Treacher Collins syndrome. Ann Plast Surg 2006;56(5):549–54.
61. Snik A, Leijendeckers J, Hol M, et al. The bone-anchored hearing aid for children: recent developments. Int J Audiol 2008;47(9):554–9.
62. Granstrom G, Tjellstrom A. The bone-anchored hearing aid (Baha) in children with auricular malformations. Ear Nose Throat J 1997;76(4):238–40, 242, 244–7.
63. Marres HA, Cremers CW, Marres EH, et al. Ear surgery in Treacher Collins syndrome. Ann Otol Rhinol Laryngol 1995;104(1):31–41.
64. Kiefer J, Arnold W, Staudenmaier R. Round window stimulation with an implantable hearing aid (Soundbridge) combined with autogenous reconstruction of the auricle—a new approach. ORL J Otorhinolaryngol Relat Spec 2006;68(6):378–85.
65. Cloonan YK, Kifle Y, Davis S, et al. Sleep outcomes in children with hemifacial microsomia and controls: a follow-up study. Pediatrics 2009;124(2):e313–21.
66. Bergmann C, Zerres K, Peschgens T, et al. Overlap between VACTERL and hemifacial microsomia illustrating a spectrum of malformations seen in axial mesodermal dysplasia complex (AMDC). Am J Med Genet A 2003;121(2):151–5.
67. Vendramini-Pittoli S, Kokitsu-Nakata NM. Oculoauriculovertebral spectrum: report of nine familial cases with evidence of autosomal dominant inheritance and review of the literature. Clin Dysmorphol 2009;18(2):67–77.
68. Balci S, Engiz O. Goldenhar syndrome and 22q11 deletion. Am J Med Genet A 2011;155:458.
69. Werler MM, Starr JR, Cloonan YK, et al. Hemifacial microsomia: from gestation to childhood. J Craniofac Surg 2009;20(1):664–9.
70. Martelli-Junior H, Teixeira de Miranda R, Moreira Fernandes C, et al. Goldenhar syndrome: clinical features with orofacial emphasis. J Appl Oral Sci 2010;18(6):646–9.
71. Anderson PJ, David DJ. Spinal anomalies in Goldenhar syndrome. Cleft Palate Craniofac J 2005;42(5):477–80.
72. Zlotogora J, Sagi M, Schuper A, et al. Variability of Stickler syndrome. Am J Med Genet 1992;42(3):337–9.
73. Vuoristo MM, Pappas JG, Jansen V, et al. A stop codon mutation in COL11A2 induces exon skippin and leand to non-ocular Stickler syndrome. Am J Med Genet A 2004;130(2):160–4.
74. Bowling EL, Brown MD, Trundle TV. The Stickler syndrome: case reports and literature review. Optometry 2000;71(3):177–82.
75. Bayazit YA, Yilmaz M. An overview of hereditary hearing loss. ORL J Otorhinolaryngol Relat Spec 2006;68(2):57–63.

Otolaryngologic Manifestations of Skeletal Dysplasias in Children

Sofia Lyford-Pike, MD[a], Julie Hoover-Fong, MD, PhD[b,c],
David E. Tunkel, MD[a,c],*

KEYWORDS

- Skeletal dysplasia • Achondroplasia • Osteogenesis imperfecta • Hearing loss
- Obstructive sleep apnea

KEY POINTS

- Children with skeletal dysplasias often present for otolaryngology evaluation; knowledge of the various syndromes and manifestations assists in diagnosis and management of ear, nose, and throat disease.
- Children with achondroplasia commonly have middle ear disease from eustachian tube dysfunction, and about half of adults and one-quarter of children with this skeletal dysplasia have hearing loss.
- Children with skeletal dysplasias are at high risk for development of obstructive sleep apnea. Although adenotonsillectomy is often the first-line treatment, the causes of sleep-disordered breathing in these patients are complex and the management is difficult.
- Children with skeletal dysplasias often undergo a variety of surgical procedures. They present unique anesthetic management issues because of variations in upper and lower airway anatomy, neck motion and stability issues, difficulties with chest and pulmonary mechanics, and abnormalities of neuromotor tone.

Skeletal dysplasias are a group of disorders of bone and cartilage development that result in abnormalities of the skeleton, with disproportionate growth of the long bones, cranium, and spine. With more than 350 types of skeletal dysplasias identified, skeletal dysplasias are estimated to affect 1 in 5000 births in the United States.[1] The most common nonlethal skeletal dysplasias are achondroplasia/hypochondroplasia, osteogenesis imperfecta (OI), variants of spondyloepiphyseal dysplasia, and

The authors have no disclosures.
[a] Department of Otolaryngology-Head and Neck Surgery, Johns Hopkins University School of Medicine, Baltimore, MD, USA; [b] Alan and Kathryn Greenberg Center for Skeletal Dysplasias, McKusick-Nathans Institute of Genetic Medicine, Johns Hopkins University School of Medicine, Baltimore, MD, USA; [c] Department of Pediatrics, Johns Hopkins University School of Medicine, Baltimore, MD, USA
* Corresponding author. Johns Hopkins Outpatient Center, Room 6161B, 601 North Caroline Street, Baltimore, MD 21287-0910.
E-mail address: dtunkel@jhmi.edu

doi:10.1016/j.otc.2012.03.002
0030-6665/12/$ – see front matter
oto.theclinics.com

pseudoachondroplasia; whereas thanatophoric dysplasia, severe OI, and achondrogenesis are common prenatal/perinatal lethal skeletal dysplasias.[2–4] Some skeletal dysplasias may be diagnosed before birth using high-resolution prenatal imaging in combination with prenatal molecular testing, but most are diagnosed at or after birth based on clinical and/or radiographic features and confirmed by molecular testing (**Table 1**).

Although skeletal dysplasias primarily manifest with short stature and orthopedic symptoms, not all are associated with short stature and many have associated otolaryngologic and even serious multisystem disease. These patients are best evaluated by a multidisciplinary team of specialists experienced in skeletal dysplasias, and head and neck manifestations of these disorders often require an otolaryngologist.

HEAD AND NECK MANIFESTATIONS

The skeletal dysplasia syndromes have a variety of head and neck manifestations. Otolaryngology evaluation of affected individuals can reveal obvious and less obvious ear, nose, and throat disease. The major issues of concern for most children with skeletal dysplasias involve the ears and hearing, and upper airway/respiratory function. An otolaryngologist experienced in the care of syndromic patients can provide specialized diagnostic services and surgical treatment of head and neck disorders associated with skeletal dysplasia. In some cases, otologic or upper airway respiratory symptoms may be the first presenting signs of these conditions.[5]

ACHONDROPLASIA

Achondroplasia is the most common syndrome of short-limb dwarfism. This autosomal dominant condition is caused by mutations in fibroblast growth factor receptor 3 (FGFR3).[6] Typical facial features include frontal bone prominence and midfacial hypoplasia, and short stature with rhizomelia is seen (**Fig. 1**). About 80% of children with achondroplasia are born to parents of average stature, indicating a new mutation in the affected child. Final height for adults with achondroplasia is slightly more than 1.2 m. Although motor delays are common in young children with achondroplasia because of macrocephaly in combination with axial and appendicular hypotonia, cognitive delays are not and require additional evaluation when identified. Almost 40% of children with achondroplasia had conductive hearing loss, and similarly 40% eventually underwent adenotonsillectomy, in one multicenter retrospective study of medical complications of achondroplasia.[7] Otolaryngologic manifestations of achondroplasia are addressed later in this article.

OTOLARYNGOLOGIC EVALUATION OF CHILDREN WITH SKELETAL DYSPLASIAS

Otolaryngologic symptoms associated with skeletal dysplasia may arise early in the neonatal period or may occur later in childhood. Otolaryngology care involves evaluation of symptomatic children with skeletal dysplasias as well as participation in routine anticipatory longitudinal medical care. The American Academy of Pediatrics Committee on Genetics has recommended, in a guideline published in 1995 and updated in 2005, that children with achondroplasia receive yearly hearing screens from infancy and undergo speech and language evaluation before 2 years of age.[8] This guideline also recommends routine screening for signs of sleep apnea, with a low threshold for testing with polysomnography and/or referral to sleep specialists. This committee suggested that such routine screening for hearing, speech, and sleep apnea is advisable in all other skeletal dysplasia diagnoses until proved to be unnecessary

Table 1
Characteristics of skeletal dysplasias

Name of Dysplasia Online Mendelian Inheritance in Man Number (omim.org)	Causative Gene Inheritance Pattern	Clinical Characteristics
Achondroplasia #100800	FGFR3 AD	Most common skeletal dysplasia. Short limbs mostly in proximal segments, macrocephaly. Midfacial hypoplasia, hypotonia, and obstructive and central apnea. Middle ear dysfunction and hearing loss common
Apert syndrome #101200	FGFR2 AD	Craniosynostosis, midfacial hypoplasia, prognathism, high-arched palate with crowded teeth, syndactyly, choanal atresia, hearing loss
Atelosteogenesis types I, II, III Types I and III #108720 Type II #256050	Type I and III FLNB AD Type II SLC26A2 AR	Atelosteogenesis is a severe disorder of cartilage and bone development. Infants born with this condition have short arms and legs, a narrow chest, and a prominent, rounded abdomen. Cleft palate, clubfeet, and hitchhiker thumbs. They are often stillborn or die soon after birth from respiratory failure. 3 variants recognized currently: types I and III caused by mutation in gene encoding filamin B, type II caused by SCL26A2 and allelic with diastrophic dysplasia
Campomelic dysplasia #114290	SOX9 AD	Severely bowed legs with disorders of the cardiac, respiratory, urinary, and central nervous systems. Manifestations include laryngotracheomalacia, micrognathia, cleft palate, low-set ears, absence of olfactory bulbs, and hypoplastic larynx
Cartilage hair hypoplasia #250250	RMRP AR	A rare form of dwarfism that is characterized by short limbs; fine, sparse hair; impaired immunity; and anemia. More common among certain ethnic groups, particularly the Amish
Chondrodysplasia punctata variants #215100, #300180, #302960	PEX7 AR ARSE X-linked	Form caused by PEX7 is rhizomelic chondrodysplasia punctata. X-linked form known as CDPX1 or caused by ARSE. CDPX2 also known as Conradi-Hunermann or Happle syndrome caused by X-linked dominant mutations in EBP. Characterized by punctate calcification of the cartilage of the epiphyses, thyroid cartilage, larynx, and trachea.

(continued on next page)

Table 1
(continued)

Name of Dysplasia Online Mendelian Inheritance in Man Number (omim.org)	Causative Gene Inheritance Pattern	Clinical Characteristics
	EBP X-linked dominant	Growth retardation, shortening of limbs, cataracts, dry and scaly skin, nasomaxillary hypoplasia, and mixed hearing loss
Cleidocranial dysplasia #119600	RUNX2 AD	Delayed or absent closure of anterior fontanelle with bulging calvaria, clavicular hypoplasia or aplasia, wide pubic symphysis, unerupted and supernumerary teeth, progressive mixed hearing loss
Diastrophic dysplasia #222600	DTDST/SLC26A2 AR	A form of dwarfism that is characterized by short limbs, cleft palate, clubfeet, hitchhiker thumb, and ears with a cauliflower appearance
Ellis-van Creveld syndrome #225500	EVC AR	Short-stature disorder characterized by short-limb dwarfism, additional fingers and/or toes, abnormal development of fingernails and teeth, and congenital heart defects. Also more common in Amish
Hypochondroplasia #146000	FGFR3 AD	Similar to achondroplasia, but features are less prominent. Often not diagnosed until 2-4 y of age
Kniest dysplasia #156550	COL2A1 AD	Individuals with Kniest dysplasia have round, flat faces with bulging and wide-set eyes. Cleft palate may be present. Tracheomalacia in some infants. Severe myopia is common, and retinal detachment is seen. Hearing loss resulting from recurrent ear infections is also possible. Similar to patients with SED(C) plus additional features of prominent joints and perhaps greater risk of retinal detachment
Larsen syndrome #150250	FLNB AD	Results from resistance to growth hormone. Characterized by prominent forehead, hypertelorism, dislocations of large joints, cleft palate, and abnormalities of the hands and feet. Laryngomalacia/tracheomalacia and subglottic stenosis have been described
Multiple epiphyseal dysplasia #132400	COMP, COL9A1, COL9A2, COL9A3, or MATN3 AD	Typically manifests later in the first decade or older with pain in hips, knees, and ankles. Mildly short stature or average stature

Disorder	Gene / Inheritance	Description
Osteogenesis imperfecta #166200, 166210, 166220, #259420	COL1A1, COL2A2 AD; CRTAP, LEPRE1, PPIB, FKBP10, SERPINH1 and SP7 AR	Disorder of abnormal type 1 collagen formation and processing, causing bone to be susceptible to fractures. May have average height but a spectrum of severity is seen. Additional signs/symptoms include blue sclera, hypermobile joints with bowing of legs and arms, and hearing loss that can be sensorineural, conductive, or mixed. Phenotypic spectrum varies from few fractures in average stature to lethal
Pseudoachondroplasia #177170	COMP AD	Often average height/length and proportionate at birth, with declining linear growth velocity by 2 y of age. Joint laxity, cervical instability
Spondyloepiphyseal dysplasia congenita #183900	COL2A1 AD	Short stature associated with hearing loss, clubfeet, cleft palate, myopia, odontoid hypoplasia, laryngotracheomalacia, and barrel chest
Stickler syndrome #108300, #604841	Type 1: COL2A1; Type 2: COL11A1; Type 3(nonocular): COL11A2; Type 4: COL9A1 AD	A progressive disorder of collagen (type I, IX, or XI), primarily associated with otologic, ocular, and orthopedic concerns. Eye concerns include myopia, retinal detachment, glaucoma, and strabismus. Other features are recurrent otitis media and sensorineural hearing loss, cleft palate often with the Pierre Robin triad, bifid uvula, flat cheeks and nasal bones, hypermobile joints, scoliosis, and osteoarthritis

Abbreviations: AD, autosomal dominant; AR, autosomal recessive; ARSE, arylsulfatase E; COL2A1, alpha1 chain of type 2 collagen; COMP, cartilage oligomeric matrix protein; DTDST, diastrophic dysplasia sulfate transporter; EBP, emopamil-binding protein; EVC, Ellis-van Creveld; FGFR3, fibroblast growth factor receptor 3 (or 2); FLNB, filamin D; PEX7, peroxisome biogenesis factor 7; RMRP, RNA component of mitochondrial RNA-processing endoribonuclease; RUNX2, runt-related transcription factor 2; SED, spondyloepiphyseal dysplasia; SOX9, SRY-BOX 9.

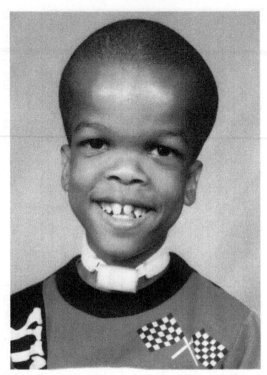

Fig. 1. Five-year-old boy with achondroplasia. He has obstructive sleep apnea so severe that he required a tracheotomy early in life. He also has hydrocephalus.

or additional diagnosis-specific recommendations are published. In addition, children with skeletal dysplasias should be followed longitudinally into adulthood for development of otolaryngologic disease such as hearing loss or sleep-disordered breathing.

Routine Evaluations

Routine otolaryngology evaluation for children with skeletal dysplasias should include a careful history directed at issues of:

- Hearing acuity
- Presence and frequency of otitis media and/or sinusitis
- Details of dynamic and static airway function.

The presence and nature of abnormal airway noises (snoring, stertor, stridor) are documented, and careful history about sleep pattern, snoring, and witnessed apneic events is elicited. Details of feeding and swallowing are discussed, and appropriate height and weight measures are documented using appropriate scales for the dysplasia diagnoses when available.[9–12] Speech and language milestones and clinical hearing assessments are an important part of this evaluation.

Craniofacial features are examined, with emphasis on:

- Nasal patency
- Size of mandible and maxilla
- Shape of palate

- Size of tongue
- Geometry of oral cavity and oropharynx.

Appearance of mucous membranes and the size of the tonsils and adenoids are documented. Otomicroscopy can be performed in the office to assess structural tympanic membrane abnormalities that may require surgical treatment. Flexible fiber-optic nasopharyngoscopy can assess nasal patency, nasopharyngeal and hypopharyngeal anatomy, supraglottic dynamics, and vocal cord motion.

Airway Evaluation for Suspected Laryngotracheal Abnormalities

When laryngotracheal abnormalities are suspected on initial evaluation, airway radiographs and/or airway endoscopy (laryngoscopy and bronchoscopy) in the operating room may be required. When severe respiratory symptoms are present, operative evaluation may occur at the time the airway is stabilized. Airway management may include endotracheal intubation, or even tracheotomy in the rare child with severe, long-standing, or multilevel airway obstruction not amenable to other treatment.

Cephalometric radiographs can quantify the abnormalities of craniofacial shape that can cause upper airway obstruction in patients with skeletal dysplasia. Computed tomography (CT) is helpful in assessing midfacial bony abnormalities such as choanal atresia, to fully assess bony sinus anatomy and presence of inflammatory sinus disease in skeletal dysplasia patients with symptoms of sinusitis, and to assess middle and inner ear anatomy through temporal bone images (**Fig. 2**).

Sleep Apnea Evaluation

Skeletal dysplasia patients with sleep-disordered breathing should be evaluated with multichannel nighttime polysomnography to document the presence and severity of sleep apnea, and to distinguish between central and obstructive apnea.[13] A recent guideline on the use of polysomnography in children before tonsillectomy

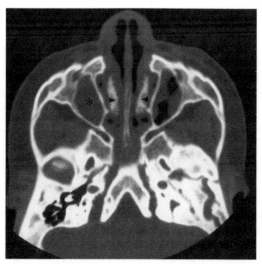

Fig. 2. Axial CT of the midfacial region in a 3-year-old patient with achondroplasia and sinusitis. Note opacification of the maxillary sinuses (*asterisk*) from sinusitis and narrowed nasal passages (*arrowheads*) associated with midfacial bony anatomy.

recommended routine use of preoperative polysomnography for children with cranio-facial anomalies.[14] This recommendation includes most, if not all, children with skeletal dysplasias who are being considered for surgical treatment of sleep-disordered breathing.

Otologic Evaluation

Patients with skeletal dysplasia and otologic disease need formal hearing assessment using pure-tone and speech audiometry. Otoscopy should evaluate common forms of middle ear disease, such as middle ear effusion, and uncommon entities such as cholesteatoma, ossicular abnormality, or high jugular bulb. When behavioral hearing tests are insufficient, objective tests such as otoacoustic emission screening and auditory brainstem response testing are used to assess hearing in uncooperative or very young patients.

AIRWAY DISORDERS ASSOCIATED WITH SKELETAL DYSPLASIA

Children with skeletal dysplasias may present with a range of respiratory signs and symptoms, from acute respiratory distress in the neonatal period to chronic concerns such as pulmonary insufficiency or sleep-associated airway obstruction. Respiratory symptoms in this population arise from multiple factors, including restrictive lung disease from abnormal thoracic anatomy, upper airway obstruction from craniofacial or pharyngeal anatomic issues, and central apneas from brainstem compression or other central nervous system abnormalities.[15]

Upper airway obstruction associated with skeletal dysplasia is usually multifactorial, with dynamic and static obstruction at multiple levels. Abnormal skull base anatomy can decrease the cross-sectional areas of the nasopharyngeal and hypopharyngeal airway. Mandibular and maxillary hypoplasia, abnormal tongue position and size, and large tonsils and adenoids can all contribute to airway narrowing at the pharyngeal level. Brachycephaly with flattening of the nasal dorsum can cause nasal airflow limitation. Associated laryngotracheal anomalies can cause fixed or dynamic narrowing of the large airways in the neck and chest, resulting in recurrent crouplike illness, stridor, and/or exercise intolerance (**Fig. 3**). Central nervous system disorders may cause poor

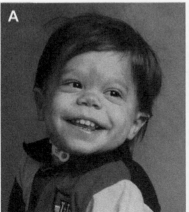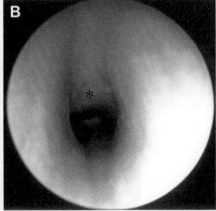

Fig. 3. (A) Toddler with skeletal dysplasia thought to be spondyloepiphyseal dysplasia, with tracheotomy for neonatal airway obstruction from subglottic stenosis. (B) Endoscopic view shows subglottic narrowing with anterior ledge from abnormal cricoid shape (*asterisk*).

pharyngeal tone or disorders of ventilatory drive that worsen the respiratory problems caused by the fixed airway obstructions.

Obstructive Sleep Apnea Syndrome in Skeletal Dysplasias

Obstructive sleep apnea syndrome (OSAS) is the most common airway disturbance seen in children with skeletal dysplasias. Children with achondroplasia are at extremely high risk for development of OSAS.[7,16] OSAS in these children may also have confounding effects on stature through the inhibition of the growth hormone axis.[17,18] Lanfranco and colleagues[18] observed a reduction in growth hormone secretion, reduced insulinlike growth factor concentration, and peripheral growth hormone insensitivity in patients with OSAS. The adverse growth effects of OSAS may be more significant for children with short-stature skeletal dysplasias.

More than 20 years ago, Reid and colleagues[19] studied 26 children with achondroplasia and found loud snoring by history in 58% and OSAS on polysomnography in 35%. Waters and colleagues[20] studied 20 patients with achondroplasia, 15 children and 5 young adults, using overnight polysomnography. All patients had evidence of upper airway obstruction on sleep study, with 75% of the studies diagnostic for OSAS.

Zucconi and colleagues[21] also diagnosed obstructive apnea and/or hypoventilation in 75% of children with achondroplasia studied with polysomnography. In addition, a recent review of 46 children with achondroplasia showed that 34.3% had sleep studies diagnostic of OSAS, of which 27.3% underwent surgical treatment, with 12.3% of those treated requiring persistent treatment with continuous positive airway pressure (CPAP).[22]

Midfacial hypoplasia, nasal and nasopharyngeal narrowing, and abnormal neural control of pharyngeal muscle tone contribute to OSAS in achondroplasia.[15,23] In 2005, Onodera and colleagues[24] compared children with OSAS with and without achondroplasia using cephalometric analysis, and the factors contributing to OSAS in children with achondroplasia were pharyngeal airway narrowing, retrognathia, increased mandibular plane angle, and increased height of the lower face.

OSAS has also been described in other skeletal dysplasias including metatropic dwarfism, Melnick-Needles syndrome, and mucopolysaccharidoses.[15,25,26] Most children with mucopolysaccharidoses (MPS) suffer from OSAS because of excessive storage of unmetabolized mucopolysaccharides. In a recent study of 24 patients using polysomnography, 22 children with the diagnoses of MPS types I, II, III, IV, and VI all had OSAS, and 88% had moderate or severe OSAS.[27] OSAS in children with MPS is attributed to the infiltration of upper airway tissues with glycosaminoglycans, in addition to tonsillar and adenoidal hypertrophy, neuromotor tone abnormalities, and craniofacial structural issues.[15] Children with MPS have a high likelihood of persistent OSAS after adenotonsillectomy.[28] In addition to palatine tonsil hypertrophy, children with MPS may have lingual tonsil hypertrophy contributing to their symptoms.[29]

Adenotonsillectomy is usually the first choice for treatment of OSAS in children, and this surgery is also used for children with skeletal dysplasias such as achondroplasia. Sisk and colleagues[30] reported that only 18% of their series of achondroplastic children with OSAS required additional treatment after adenotonsillectomy, whereas 90% of the children who had adenoidectomy alone required additional surgery. Adenotonsillectomy was reported to help relieve pulmonary hypertension in a 5-year-old child with achondroplasia and severe OSAS.[31]

Pearls and *Pitfalls: Patients with craniofacial abnormalities are at high risk for respiratory compromise after adenotonsillectomy, and postoperative cardiorespiratory monitoring in an inpatient setting is mandatory for such patients.*[32–34]

Postoperative polysomnography is recommended after adenotonsillectomy for OSAS in children with skeletal dysplasias, because OSAS often persists.[22,35] Patients with persistent OSAS after adenotonsillectomy can be considered for additional surgery based on specific anatomic issues:

- Turbinate reduction
- Uvulopalatopharyngoplasty[36]
- Tongue resection
- Tracheotomy.[15,37]

Craniofacial reconstructive techniques involving mandibular and midfacial advancement and maxillary expansion may improve OSAS in patients with the craniofacial abnormalities seen in skeletal dysplasias.[38,39] Successful decannulation of patients with tracheostomy was achieved in 2 young children with achondroplasia using midface distraction osteogenesis procedures.[40] CPAP or bilevel positive airway pressure (BiPAP) are nonsurgical treatments of OSAS in complex patients, when OSAS persists after adenotonsillectomy or other surgery or when surgery is contraindicated.[15] Waters and colleagues[35] studied achondroplastic patients with OSAS, 13 of whom were treated with CPAP, and found improvement in polysomnographic measures and, for some cases, improvement in measured somatosensory evoked potentials. Although CPAP or BiPAP are effective treatments of OSAS in complex sleep-related airway obstruction, difficulties with compliance are magnified in young children.

Central apnea is also seen in children with achondroplasia. Children with achondroplasia may have foramen magnum stenosis and/or hydrocephalus.[41] Brainstem compression at the craniocervical junction has been implicated in abnormal airway control seen in these patients. It is thought that this may be a contributing factor to sudden infant death, which occurs in 2% to 5% of these children.[19,42] Physicians are encouraged to actively screen patients for this anomaly.[8] Infants with achondroplasia should undergo assessment for craniocervical junction abnormalities, an assessment that often includes careful neurologic history and examination, neuroimaging, and polysomnography.[43] When such compression is identified, surgical decompression of the posterior fossa has improved respiratory function.[44,45] Although in one small retrospective series up to 50% of patients required decompression of foramen magnum stenosis, a recent review suggests that 5% to 10% of achondroplastic patients require this neurosurgical intervention.[46,47]

Laryngotracheal Abnormalities in Skeletal Dysplasias

Abnormalities of the larynx and trachea have been associated with specific skeletal dysplasia diagnoses. Myer and Cotton[48] described 2 patients with spondyloepiphyseal dysplasia (SED), an autosomal dominant skeletal dysplasia arising from a mutation affecting collagen II production, who each required tracheotomy for subglottic stenosis. One of the patients with SED had glottic and supraglottic abnormalities in addition to the stenosis below the vocal cords. One patient underwent laryngotracheal reconstruction using a costal cartilage graft, but remained tracheotomy dependent despite surgical efforts.

We have treated 2 such patients with SED and subglottic stenosis requiring tracheotomy in infancy. One underwent costal cartilage graft laryngotracheal reconstruction, but was not decannulated until 4 years after surgery. Another child with SED and congenital subglottic stenosis was decannulated from tracheotomy at age 7 years without surgical intervention.

Myer and Cotton[48] caution that intrinsic cartilage abnormalities in such skeletal dysplasias may compromise the results of standard techniques of augmentation/ repair of laryngeal stenosis, which rely on the use of rigid cartilage grafts to restore laryngeal lumen size and framework rigidity.[48]

Long-segment tracheobronchial stenosis has been described in patients with chondrodysplasia punctata, a group of heterogeneous skeletal disorders characterized by punctiform calcifications of bone, in which lengthy areas of tracheal narrowing are associated cartilage calcifications (**Fig. 4**).[49] Larsen syndrome is a rare skeletal dysplasia characterized by:

- Prominent forehead.
- Hypertelorism.
- Dislocations of large joints.
- Abnormalities of the hands and feet.
- Laryngomalacia and tracheomalacia have been described in infants.[50,51]
- Congenital subglottic stenosis has been described in 3 patients, all of whom required tracheotomy early in life.[52] These patients were successfully treated by cricotracheal resection with primary anastomosis after failure of augmentation laryngotracheal reconstruction.

Some skeletal dysplasias may also result in structurally deficient laryngeal and/or tracheal cartilage. Infants with campomelic dysplasia, a skeletal dysplasia caused by mutations in or near the SOX9 gene, can have severe respiratory difficulties both from Pierre Robin–like retrognathia and glossoptosis as well as from diffuse laryngotracheobronchomalacia secondary to faulty cartilaginous support. Grad and colleagues[53] described bronchoscopic findings of severe fixed and dynamic airway compromise that led to respiratory failure in 2 children, even after tracheotomy in 1

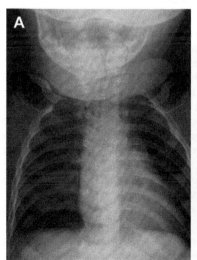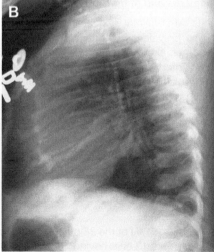

Fig. 4. Tracheal stenosis and associated tracheal cartilage calcifications seen on (A) anteroposterior and (B) lateral views of chest radiographs of a child with chondrodysplasia punctata.

infant. Ruan and colleagues[54] successfully treated a 2-year-old child with campomelic dysplasia and laryngotracheomalacia with an anterior laryngotracheal reconstruction using a long costal graft that extended from the thyroid cartilage to the seventh tracheal ring.

Severe tracheomalacia has been seen in association with the thoracic (rib and vertebral) abnormalities seen in spondylothoracic or spondylocostal dysostosis, previously referred to as Jarcho-Levin syndrome. Tracheal stenting has been described in such cases, but should be considered only for life-threatening airway obstruction not amenable to other treatment, because fatal complications of such stents have been reported.[55]

Nasal Abnormalities Associated with Skeletal Dysplasias

Nasal obstruction associated with skeletal dysplasia syndromes can occur from craniofacial structural abnormalities with reduced nasal and nasopharyngeal airway size, or from discrete obstructive lesions associated with the syndrome. Patients with achondroplasia have shortened cranial base length and a more acute cranial base angle.[56] Recessed maxilla, reduced facial height, and depressed nasal bones all contribute to nasal airflow limitations.

Choanal atresia has been reported in 1 child with achondroplasia, and has been associated with a variety of other syndromes with craniofacial anomalies (eg, Apert syndrome, CHARGE [coloboma, central nervous system anomalies, heart defects, atresia of the choanae, retardation of growth and/or development, ear anomalies and/or deafness] association)[57] In addition, nasomaxillary hypoplasia with reduced nasal airway flow is a common feature of chondrodysplasia punctata.[49,58] Choanal stenosis was also described in craniometaphyseal and craniodiaphyseal dysplasia, and surgical intervention for stenosis provided little benefit in these progressive disorders.[59]

OTOLOGIC MANIFESTATIONS OF SKELETAL DYSPLASIA
Hearing Loss and Middle Ear Disease in Patients with Skeletal Dysplasia

Patients with Skeletal dysplasia can have conductive, sensorineural, or mixed hearing loss. The prevalence of hearing loss in children with achondroplasia, and perhaps some other skeletal dysplasia diagnoses, supports routine testing of hearing at frequent intervals in affected children.[8] Conductive hearing loss in children with achondroplasia is often from middle ear dysfunction, and tympanostomy tube placement can improve hearing loss. Some patients with ossicular abnormalities associated with skeletal dysplasias may be amenable to ossiculoplasty or stapedectomy. Amplification with hearing aids should be considered for persistent conductive hearing loss in children that does not respond to management of middle ear disease, or for those with sensorineural hearing loss.

The frequency of hearing abnormalities associated with skeletal dysplasia was shown by Glass and colleagues,[60] who performed hearing evaluation in 38 patients with skeletal dysplasia. Of these, 28 had achondroplasia, and 27 were 20 years old or younger.

Seventeen (61%) of the 28 patients with achondroplasia had hearing loss in at least 1 ear, with 13 ears having conductive loss, 7 ears having sensorineural loss, and 1 ear having a mixed loss.

Only 20% of the patients with skeletal dysplasia diagnoses other than achondroplasia had hearing loss in this series.

Stura and colleagues[61] tested hearing in patients with skeletal dysplasias, all aged 21 years or younger.

55% of the achondroplasia had hearing loss, two-thirds had conductive hearing loss, and one-third had sensorineural hearing loss.

Similarly, only 20% of the patients with skeletal dysplasias other than achondroplasia had hearing loss in this report.

Middle ear disease is seen in most children with achondroplasia. Berkowitz and colleagues[56] reviewed the charts of 61 young patients with achondroplasia and found that 54% had a history of tympanostomy tube insertion.

Four of these patients had tympanic membrane perforations
One had a cholesteatoma
One had ossicular chain erosion.

Collins and Choi[47] reviewed 22 patients with achondroplasia, and found documented otologic disease in 68% and hearing loss in 68%. Notably, there was no record of hearing aid use for any patient.

In 1988, Cobb and colleagues[62] compared CT scans of the temporal bones of 9 patients with achondroplasia with the scans of 10 nonsyndromic patients. They described:

Poor mastoid pneumatization
Shortening of the carotid canals
Skull base narrowing
Towering petrous ridges
Rotation of the cochlea leading to the abnormal relative orientation of the inner ear, middle ear, and external auditory canal.[62]

Further evaluation of high-resolution CT scans of the temporal bones in 9 patients with achondroplasia found no correlation between anatomic findings and degree of hearing loss.[63]

Jugular bulb dehiscence in the middle ear was described more than 35 years ago in 2 patients with skeletal dysplasia.[64] Pauli and Modaff[65] found such jugular bulb anomalies in 3% of a large group of patients with achondroplasia, manifested by conductive hearing loss and/or pulsatile tinnitus.

PEARLS and PITFALLS: The association of jugular bulb dehiscence with achondroplasia merits caution during myringotomy procedures for middle ear effusion in these patients (Fig. 5).

A recent hearing screening program at a 2010 convention of individuals with short-stature skeletal dysplasias identified hearing loss in 1 or both ears in at least one-quarter of children tested, and middle ear dysfunction as identified by abnormal tympanometry in more than one-half of tested children (**Fig. 6**).[66]

Three-quarters of the children tested had achondroplasia. Hearing loss was not suspected in many of the individuals who failed hearing screening. It is clear that children with skeletal dysplasia require regular objective hearing assessments and careful ear examinations, with intervention when hearing loss and/or middle ear disease is identified.

Many of the various skeletal dysplasia syndromes besides achondroplasia have otologic manifestations including hearing loss. Dahiya and colleagues[67] reported that 25% to 30% of patients with SED have hearing loss that is usually sensorineural,

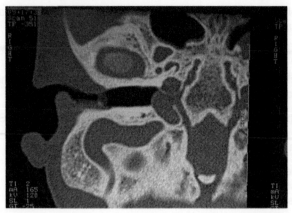

Fig. 5. Axial CT of the temporal bone of a patient with achondroplasia. Note that the right middle ear is filled with a high dehiscent jugular bulb touching the tympanic membrane.

although a conductive component is also seen in SED, a dysplasia caused by abnormal type II collagen. Most patients with diastrophic dysplasia, an autosomal recessive short-stature syndrome, develop cystic swellings of the pinna in infancy that usually progress to hard cauliflower-type auricular deformities.[68] These patients can also develop stenotic ear canals. In our 2010 hearing screening study, hearing loss was identified in several children with spondyloepiphyseal dysplasia, cartilage hair hypoplasia, and Morquio syndrome (mucopolysaccharidosis type IV).

Thirty-three percent of patients with cleidocranial dysplasia, an autosomal dominant skeletal dysplasia manifested by open skull sutures and clavicular hypoplasia or aplasia, were found to have conductive, sensorineural or mixed hearing loss.[69] For this dysplasia, caused by a mutation in the osteoblast-specific transcription factor CBFA1, hearing loss may be the presenting symptom that leads to syndromic diagnosis.[5]

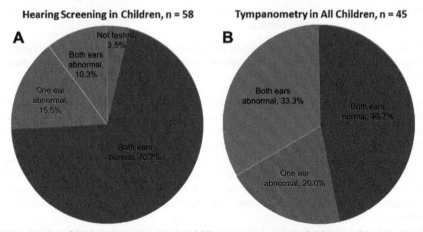

Fig. 6. Results of (A) hearing screening and (B) tympanometry in children at the Little People of America convention in 2010. More than one-quarter of the children had hearing loss in at least 1 ear, and more than one-half had evidence of middle ear dysfunction.

OI and Hearing Loss

Hearing loss is seen in many patients with OI, a group of disorders of collagen 1 synthesis and processing, manifested most notably with bone fragility. OI is classically inherited in an autosomal dominant pattern with mutations in *COL1A1* and *COL1A2*, but several recessive forms have also been described with mutations in *CRTAP*, *LEPRE1*, *PPIB*, *FKBP10*, *SERPINH1*, and *SP7*. Disease severity in OI ranges from lethal forms to disease manifested by mild bony involvement and hearing loss. Pillion and Shapiro[70] found hearing loss in 37% to 78% of these patients.[70,71] The hearing loss associated with OI becomes more frequent and more severe with age[70]:

- 31% of patients less than 10 years of age
- 95% of patients more than 30 years of age.

Mixed hearing losses with a large conductive component are most common, seen in 51% of the patients with OI with hearing loss. Quisling and colleagues[72] studied 160 family members of a single patient with OI, and 47% had hearing loss, 66% had fragile bones, and 56% had blue sclera.

The conductive hearing loss of OI is often from otitis media with effusion in younger patients. With advancing age, ossicular dysfunction plays a larger role in loss of hearing.[70] An otosclerosislike process with deposition of abnormal bone around the stapes footplate causes ossicular chain fixation. Fibrous degeneration of the stapes crura has also been seen in some surgical cases and in temporal bone specimens. OI-associated hearing loss occurs earlier than that of otosclerosis, and is usually clinically apparent in the second or third decades of life. Middle ear involvement tends to be more severe in OI, and more patients (up to 41%) have sensorineural hearing loss in addition to conductive hearing loss.[70,73]

Stapes surgery for OI and hearing loss

Although amplification with hearing aids should be the first intervention for children with OI and hearing loss (not from middle ear effusion), stapes surgery can improve hearing in older patients with conductive hearing loss. The findings at middle ear exploration of patients with OI with conductive hearing loss are fixation of the stapes footplate with immature-appearing, chalky, soft, vascular bony deposits, and, less frequently, fracture and resorption of the stapes suprastructure.[74] Shea and Postma[75] reported improved hearing at 1-year follow-up in 84% of 51 patients with OI undergoing stapedectomy. Seventy-five percent of patients had complete resolution of the conductive component of hearing loss after surgery. More recent series confirmed improvement with stapes surgery in this population.[76] Swinnen and colleagues[77] followed 12 patients with OI who underwent stapes surgery, and showed that, of the 13 ears operated, 12 had long-term reduction of the preoperative air-bone gap.

Stapes surgery for OI-associated conductive hearing loss has more potential complications than similar surgery done for otosclerosis. The tympanic ring may fracture during curetting or drilling, the stapes crura can be inadvertently fractured, the stapes footplate can become excessively mobile during drilling, and the long process of the incus can be crushed when the stapes prosthesis is applied.[78] Troublesome bleeding may obscure microscopic visualization as well.[73,75]

Cochlear implantation for OI and hearing loss

Cochlear implantation has been advocated for patients with OI with severe sensorineural hearing loss. Two reports have documented the feasibility and benefits of cochlear implantation for patients with OI.[79] Preoperative temporal bone CT scans are necessary to rule out associated anatomic aberrations that could impede implantation. One of the 3 cases reported by Rotteveel and colleagues[80] had misplacement of the electrode array into the horizontal semicircular canal at surgery.

ANESTHETIC AND PERIOPERATIVE CONSIDERATIONS FOR CHILDREN WITH SKELETAL DYSPLASIAS

The otolaryngologist may be involved in anesthetics given the frequency for routine otolaryngologic surgical procedures such as adenotonsillectomy and/or tympanostomy tube placement in these children. In addition, an otolaryngologist may be asked to assist with airway management on induction or emergence from anesthesia for syndromic children with complex airway disorders when they are undergoing other surgery, such as orthopedic or neurosurgical procedures. The Medical Advisory Board of the Little People of America has provided suggestions for the anesthesia care and preoperative assessment of individuals with skeletal dysplasias, available at www.lpaonline.org.

PEARLS and PITFALLS: *There are several important considerations for safe anesthesia for children with skeletal dysplasias.*

Even the usually simple task of establishing venous access may be challenging in a child with limb abnormalities from a skeletal dysplasia. Medication dosing is performed based on body weight, rather than by age or height. Patient positioning may be problematic because some patients with certain skeletal dysplasias have difficulty laying supine because of both obstructive airway symptoms and costovertebral malformations.[81] Forced hyperextension of the neck should be avoided during direct laryngoscopy/endotracheal intubation because cervical spinal cord compression could occur.[30] Cervical spine abnormalities can be present in many skeletal dysplasias, but can be most significant in patients with SED, Morquio syndrome (MPS IV), and pseudoachondroplasia who may have atlantoaxial instability.[82] Fifty-three percent of patients with achondroplasia require a smaller endotracheal tube than that predicted by age-based formulas.

Children with skeletal dysplasias can have airway obstruction and restrictive pulmonary issues, and it should be expected that these respiratory difficulties will be even more significant during an operative procedure. Bag-mask ventilation may be impaired by craniofacial anomalies, small nasal air passages, macroglossia, or glossoptosis. Airway management may involve a host of resources, such as fiber-optic intubation for patients with neck instability or rigid bronchoscopy for children suspected to have laryngotracheal lesions. The otolaryngologist can anticipate these issues with a thorough knowledge of the airway manifestations of a given skeletal dysplasia diagnosis, a multidisciplinary assessment before surgery, and communication of these details with the anesthesiologist.

The otolaryngologist should also participate in postoperative care for patients with skeletal dysplasia and known difficulties in airway management. The decision to perform tracheotomy in a child with complex airway issues is never simple, but should include considerations of the need for long-term airway support after the procedure, the anticipated difficulties in reestablishing airway control if needed, and the available resources and skills in the postoperative care environment.

REFERENCES

1. Krakow D, Rimoin DL. The skeletal dysplasias. Genet Med 2010;12(6):327–41.

2. Orioli IM, Castilla EE, Barbosa-Neto JG. The birth prevalence rates for the skeletal dysplasias. J Med Genet 1986;23(4):328–32.
3. Schild RL, Hunt GH, Moore J, et al. Antenatal sonographic diagnosis of thanatophoric dysplasia: a report of three cases and a review of the literature with special emphasis on the differential diagnosis. Ultrasound Obstet Gynecol 1996;8(1):62–7.
4. Superti-Furga A, Hastbacka J, Wilcox WR, et al. Achondrogenesis type IB is caused by mutations in the diastrophic dysplasia sulphate transporter gene. Nat Genet 1996;12(1):100–2.
5. Dhooge I, Lantsoght B, Lemmerling M, et al. Hearing loss as a presenting symptom of cleidocranial dysplasia. Otol Neurotol 2001;22(6):855–7.
6. He L, Shobnam N, Wimley WC, et al. FGFR3 heterodimerization in achondroplasia, the most common form of human dwarfism. J Biol Chem 2011;286(15):13272–81.
7. Hunter AG, Bankier A, Rogers JG, et al. Medical complications of achondroplasia: a multicentre patient review. J Med Genet 1998;35(9):705–12.
8. Trotter TL, Hall JG. Health supervision for children with achondroplasia. Pediatrics 2005;116(3):771–83.
9. Hoover-Fong JE, McGready J, Schulze KJ, et al. Weight for age charts for children with achondroplasia. Am J Med Genet A 2007;143(19):2227–35.
10. Horton WA, Hall JG, Scott CI, et al. Growth curves for height for diastrophic dysplasia, spondyloepiphyseal dysplasia congenita, and pseudoachondroplasia. Am J Dis Child 1982;136(4):316–9.
11. Horton WA, Rotter JI, Rimoin DL, et al. Standard growth curves for achondroplasia. J Pediatr 1978;93(3):435–8.
12. Hoover-Fong JE, Schulze KJ, McGready J, et al. Age-appropriate body mass index in children with achondroplasia: interpretation in relation to indexes of height. Am J Clin Nutr 2008;88(2):364–71.
13. Sterni LM, Tunkel DE. Obstructive sleep apnea in children: an update. Pediatr Clin North Am 2003;50(2):427–43.
14. Roland PS, Rosenfeld RM, Brooks LJ, et al. Clinical practice guideline: polysomnography for sleep-disordered breathing prior to tonsillectomy in children. Otolaryngol Head Neck Surg 2011;145(Suppl 1):S1–15.
15. Mogayzel PJ, Marcus CL. Skeletal dysplasias and their effect on the respiratory system. Paediatr Respir Rev 2001;2(4):365–71.
16. Carter EM, Davis JG, Raggio CL. Advances in understanding etiology of achondroplasia and review of management. Curr Opin Pediatr 2007;19(1):32–7.
17. Onodera K, Sakata H, Niikuni N, et al. Survey of the present status of sleep-disordered breathing in children with achondroplasia. Part I. A questionnaire survey. Int J Pediatr Otorhinolaryngol 2005;69(4):457–61.
18. Lanfranco F, Motta G, Minetto MA, et al. Growth hormone/insulin-like growth factor-I axis in obstructive sleep apnea syndrome: an update. J Endocrinol Invest 2010;33(3):192–6.
19. Reid CS, Pyeritz RE, Kopits SE, et al. Cervicomedullary compression in young patients with achondroplasia: value of comprehensive neurologic and respiratory evaluation. J Pediatr 1987;110(4):522–30.
20. Waters KA, Everett F, Sillence D, et al. Breathing abnormalities in sleep in achondroplasia. Arch Dis Child 1993;69(2):191–6.
21. Zucconi M, Weber G, Castronovo V, et al. Sleep and upper airway obstruction in children with achondroplasia. J Pediatr 1996;129(5):743–9.
22. Afsharpaiman S, Sillence DO, Sheikhvatan M, et al. Respiratory events and obstructive sleep apnea in children with achondroplasia: investigation and treatment outcomes. Sleep Breath 2011;15(4):755–61.

23. Carroll JL, McColley SA, Marcus CL, et al. Inability of clinical history to distinguish primary snoring from obstructive sleep apnea syndrome in children. Chest 1995; 108(3):610–8.

24. Onodera K, Niikuni N, Chigono T, et al. Sleep disordered breathing in children with achondroplasia. Part 2. Relationship with craniofacial and airway morphology. Int J Pediatr Otorhinolaryngol 2006;70(3):453–61.

25. Belik J, Anday EK, Kaplan F, et al. Respiratory complications of metatropic dwarfism. Clin Pediatr (Phila) 1985;24(9):504–11.

26. Molina FM, Morales C, Taylor JA. Mandibular distraction osteogenesis in a patient with Melnick-Needles syndrome. J Craniofac Surg 2008;19(1):277–9.

27. Lin HY, Chen MR, Lin CC, et al. Polysomnographic characteristics in patients with mucopolysaccharidoses. Pediatr Pulmonol 2010;45(12):1205–12.

28. Santos S, Lopez L, Gonzalez L, et al. Hearing loss and airway problems in children with mucopolysaccharidoses. Acta Otorrinolaringol Esp 2011;62(6):411–7.

29. Abdel-Aziz M, Ibrahim N, Ahmed A, et al. Lingual tonsils hypertrophy; a cause of obstructive sleep apnea in children after adenotonsillectomy: operative problems and management. Int J Pediatr Otorhinolaryngol 2011;75(9):1127–31.

30. Sisk EA, Heatley DG, Borowski BJ, et al. Obstructive sleep apnea in children with achondroplasia: surgical and anesthetic considerations. Otolaryngol Head Neck Surg 1999;120(2):248–54.

31. Yildirim SV, Durmaz C, Pourbagher MA, et al. A case of achondroplasia with severe pulmonary hypertension due to obstructive sleep apnea. Eur Arch Otorhinolaryngol 2006;263(8):775–7.

32. McColley SA, April MM, Carroll JL, et al. Respiratory compromise after adenotonsillectomy in children with obstructive sleep apnea. Arch Otolaryngol Head Neck Surg 1992;118(9):940–3.

33. Rosen GM, Muckle RP, Mahowald MW, et al. Postoperative respiratory compromise in children with obstructive sleep apnea syndrome: can it be anticipated? Pediatrics 1994;93(5):784–8.

34. Biavati MJ, Manning SC, Phillips DL. Predictive factors for respiratory complications after tonsillectomy and adenoidectomy in children. Arch Otolaryngol Head Neck Surg 1997;123(5):517–21.

35. Waters KA, Everett F, Sillence DO, et al. Treatment of obstructive sleep apnea in achondroplasia: evaluation of sleep, breathing, and somatosensory-evoked potentials. Am J Med Genet 1995;59(4):460–6.

36. Kosko JR, Derkay CS. Uvulopalatopharyngoplasty: treatment of obstructive sleep apnea in neurologically impaired pediatric patients. Int J Pediatr Otorhinolaryngol 1995;32(3):241–6.

37. Tunkel DE, McColley SA, Baroody FM, et al. Polysomnography in the evaluation of readiness for decannulation in children. Arch Otolaryngol Head Neck Surg 1996; 122(7):721–4.

38. Burstein FD, Cohen SR, Scott PH, et al. Surgical therapy for severe refractory sleep apnea in infants and children: application of the airway zone concept. Plast Reconstr Surg 1995;96(1):34–41.

39. James D, Ma L. Mandibular reconstruction in children with obstructive sleep apnea due to micrognathia. Plast Reconstr Surg 1997;100(5):1131–7 [discussion: 1138].

40. Elwood ET, Burstein FD, Graham L, et al. Midface distraction to alleviate upper airway obstruction in achondroplastic dwarfs. Cleft Palate Craniofac J 2003; 40(1):100–3.

41. King JA, Vachhrajani S, Drake JM, et al. Neurosurgical implications of achondroplasia. J Neurosurg Pediatr 2009;4(4):297–306.

42. Pauli RM, Scott CI, Wassman ER Jr, et al. Apnea and sudden unexpected death in infants with achondroplasia. J Pediatr 1984;104(3):342–8.
43. Pauli RM, Horton VK, Glinski LP, et al. Prospective assessment of risks for cervicomedullary-junction compression in infants with achondroplasia. Am J Hum Genet 1995;56(3):732–44.
44. Nelson FW, Hecht JT, Horton WA, et al. Neurological basis of respiratory complications in achondroplasia. Ann Neurol 1988;24(1):89–93.
45. Bagley CA, Pindrik JA, Bookland MJ, et al. Cervicomedullary decompression for foramen magnum stenosis in achondroplasia. J Neurosurg 2006;104(Suppl 3): 166–72.
46. Horton WA, Hall JG, Hecht JT. Achondroplasia. Lancet 2007;370(9582):162–72.
47. Collins WO, Choi SS. Otolaryngologic manifestations of achondroplasia. Arch Otolaryngol Head Neck Surg 2007;133(3):237–44.
48. Myer CM 3rd, Cotton RT. Laryngotracheal stenosis in spondyloepiphyseal dysplasia. Laryngoscope 1985;95(1):3–5.
49. Wolpoe ME, Braverman N, Lin SY. Severe tracheobronchial stenosis in the X-linked recessive form of chondrodysplasia punctata. Arch Otolaryngol Head Neck Surg 2004;130(12):1423–6.
50. Latta RJ, Graham CB, Aase J, et al. Larsen's syndrome: a skeletal dysplasia with multiple joint dislocations and unusual facies. J Pediatr 1971;78(2):291–8.
51. Grundfast KM, Mumtaz A, Kanter R, et al. Tracheomalacia in an infant with multiplex congenita (Larsen's) syndrome. Ann Otol Rhinol Laryngol 1981;90(4 Pt 1):303–6.
52. Hoeve HJ, Joosten KF, Bogers AJ, et al. Malformation and stenosis of the cricoid cartilage in association with Larsen's syndrome. Laryngoscope 1997;107(6): 792–4.
53. Grad R, Sammut PH, Britton JR, et al. Bronchoscopic evaluation of airway obstruction in campomelic dysplasia. Pediatr Pulmonol 1987;3(5):364–7.
54. Ruan L, Mitchell RB, Pereira KD, et al. Campomelic syndrome–laryngotracheomalacia treated with single-stage laryngotracheal reconstruction. Int J Pediatr Otorhinolaryngol 1996;37(3):277–81.
55. Stotz WH, Berkowitz ID, Hoehner JC, et al. Fatal complication from a balloon-expandable tracheal stent in a child: a case report. Pediatr Crit Care Med 2003;4(1):115–7.
56. Berkowitz RG, Grundfast KM, Scott C, et al. Middle ear disease in childhood achondroplasia. Ear Nose Throat J 1991;70(5):305–8.
57. Oestreich AE. Choanal atresia with achondroplasia. J Pediatr 1980;96(2):343–4.
58. Webster HR, Marshall DR. Nasal augmentation in chondrodysplasia punctata using tissue expansion. Br J Plast Surg 1991;44(5):384–5.
59. Richards A, Brain C, Dillon MJ, et al. Craniometaphyseal and craniodiaphyseal dysplasia, head and neck manifestations and management. J Laryngol Otol 1996;110(4):328–38.
60. Glass L, Shapiro I, Hodge SE, et al. Audiological findings of patients with achondroplasia. Int J Pediatr Otorhinolaryngol 1981;3(2):129–35.
61. Stura M, Boero S, Origo C, et al. Evaluation of hearing in achondroplastic patients. Basic Life Sci 1988;48:183–6.
62. Cobb SR, Shohat M, Mehringer CM, et al. CT of the temporal bone in achondroplasia. AJNR Am J Neuroradiol 1988;9(6):1195–9.
63. Shohat M, Flaum E, Cobb SR, et al. Hearing loss and temporal bone structure in achondroplasia. Am J Med Genet 1993;45(5):548–51.
64. West JM, Bandy BC, Jafek BW. Aberrant jugular bulb in the middle ear cavity. Arch Otolaryngol 1974;100(5):370–2.

65. Pauli RM, Modaff P. Jugular bulb dehiscence in achondroplasia. Int J Pediatr Oto-rhinolaryngol 1999;48(2):169–74.
66. Tunkel DE, Kerbavaz R, Smith B, et al. Hearing screening in children with skeletal dysplasia. Arch Otolaryngol Head Neck Surg 2011;137(12):1236–9.
67. Dahiya R, Cleveland S, Megerian CA. Spondyloepiphyseal dysplasia congenita associated with conductive hearing loss. Ear Nose Throat J 2000;79(3):178–82.
68. Walker BA, Scott CI, Hall JG, et al. Diastrophic dwarfism. Medicine (Baltimore) 1972;51(1):41–59.
69. Visosky AM, Johnson J, Bingea B, et al. Otolaryngological manifestations of cleidocranial dysplasia, concentrating on audiological findings. Laryngoscope 2003; 113(9):1508–14.
70. Pillion JP, Shapiro J. Audiological findings in osteogenesis imperfecta. J Am Acad Audiol 2008;19(8):595–601.
71. Garretsen AJ, Cremers CW, Huygen PL. Hearing loss (in nonoperated ears) in relation to age in osteogenesis imperfecta type I. Ann Otol Rhinol Laryngol 1997;106(7 Pt 1):575–82.
72. Quisling RW, Moore GR, Jahrsdoerfer RA, et al. Osteogenesis imperfecta. A study of 160 family members. Arch Otolaryngol 1979;105(4):207–11.
73. Cohen BJ. Osteogenesis imperfecta and hearing loss. Ear Nose Throat J 1984; 63(6):283–8.
74. Patterson CN, Stone HB 3rd. Stapedectomy in Van der Hoeve's syndrome. Laryngoscope 1970;80(4):544–58.
75. Shea JJ, Postma DS. Findings and long-term surgical results in the hearing loss of osteogenesis imperfecta. Arch Otolaryngol 1982;108(8):467–70.
76. Kuurila K, Pynnonen S, Grenman R. Stapes surgery in osteogenesis imperfecta in Finland. Ann Otol Rhinol Laryngol 2004;113(3 Pt 1):187–93.
77. Swinnen FK, De Leenheer EM, Coucke PJ, et al. Audiometric, surgical, and genetic findings in 15 ears of patients with osteogenesis imperfecta. Laryngoscope 2009;119(6):1171–9.
78. Kosoy J, Maddox HE 3rd. Surgical findings in van der Hoeve's syndrome. Arch Otolaryngol 1971;93(2):115–22.
79. Streubel SO, Lustig LR. Cochlear implantation in patients with osteogenesis imperfecta. Otolaryngol Head Neck Surg 2005;132(5):735–40.
80. Rotteveel LJ, Beynon AJ, Mens LH, et al. Cochlear implantation in 3 patients with osteogenesis imperfecta: imaging, surgery and programming issues. Audiol Neurootol 2008;13(2):73–85.
81. Krishnan BS, Eipe N, Korula G. Anaesthetic management of a patient with achondroplasia. Paediatr Anaesth 2003;13(6):547–9.
82. Berkowitz ID, Raja SN, Bender KS, et al. Dwarfs: pathophysiology and anesthetic implications. Anesthesiology 1990;73(4):739–59.

The Otolaryngologist's Approach to the Patient with Down Syndrome

Regina Rodman, MD*, Harold S. Pine, MD

KEYWORDS

- Otolaryngology • Down syndrome • Quality of life • Morphology • Otitis media
- Hearing loss • Obstructive sleep apnea • Tonsillectomy • Sinusitis • Intubation
- Acquired subglottic stenosis

KEY POINTS

- The child with Down syndrome should undergo behavioral audiologic testing every 6 months, or every 3 months if the patient has very stenotic ear canals. Treatment of hearing loss caused by recurrent otitis media and otitis media with effusion (OME) should be aggressive, with close follow-up. Parents should be prepared for multiple sets of pressure equalization (PE) tubes throughout the child's life.
- Up to 80% of patients with Down syndrome have obstructive sleep apnea. All children with Down syndrome should get an overnight polysomnography study between the ages of 3 and 4 years. Parents are not reliable in assessing sleep apnea.
- Primary treatment of obstructive sleep apnea syndrome (OSAS) is tonsillectomy and adenoidectomy, but parents should be prepared that this is curative in only 25% to 50% of children with Down syndrome, and that their child may require further surgery to alleviate obstruction, or the child may continue to require continuous positive airway pressure (CPAP).
- Airway anomalies are more common in the Down syndrome population, including subglottic stenosis. Prevention of subglottic stenosis can be achieved in part by using an endotracheal tube 2 sizes smaller than predicted for the patient's age, and ensuring that an audible air leak is present around the tube.
- During surgery in patients with Down syndrome, the surgeon should always be aware of the possibility of atlantoaxial instability, and no dramatic head movement should be made.

Conflict of interest: Neither Harold Pine, MD, nor Regina Rodman, MD, has any conflict of interest that pertains to this paper. Dr Harold Pine serves on the advisory board for Arthrocare Corporation.
Department of Otolaryngology, University of Texas Medical Branch, 301 University Boulevard, Galveston, TX 77555, USA
* Corresponding author.
E-mail address: reginarodman@yahoo.com

DOWN SYNDROME

A syndrome is a collection of features that occur together and make up a characteristic clinical entity. In 1886, John Landon Down described the syndrome including microgenia (round face), macroglossia, epicanthal folds, upslanting palpebral fissures, shorter limbs, a single transverse palmar crease, poor muscle tone, mental retardation, and learning disabilities.

The condition was identified as a chromosome 21 trisomy by Jérôme Lejeune in 1959. Today, Down syndrome is the most common congenital chromosome anomaly, occurring in 1 of 700 live births.[1] Recent advances in surgery for the treatment of congenital heart defects have greatly enhanced the survival of children with Down syndrome.[2] Although life expectancy among persons with Down syndrome remains decreased relative to the general population, studies in developed countries document sizable gains in child survival, from 25 years in 1983[3] to an estimated life expectancy of 50 to 60 years today.[4] As more of these patients are living into adulthood, attention has been focused on health factors that affect the quality of patients' lives, and affect their ability to reach full potential. A survey of parents attending a Down Syndrome Association conference showed that 50% of children with Down syndrome saw an otolaryngologist regularly.[5] It is likely that the practicing otolaryngologist will encounter many children with Down syndrome, and appropriate treatment can have a significant impact on the quality of life of these patients.

Patients with Down syndrome have several morphologic abnormalities that predispose them to problems with the ear, nose and throat. They have midface hypoplasia with malformation of the eustachian tube,[6] leading to an increased number of ear infections and hearing loss, much of which is preventable with aggressive intervention. They also have shortened palate,[7] relative macroglossia, narrowing of the oropharynx and nasopharynx,[8] and generalized hypotonia, which greatly increases the frequency and severity of obstructive sleep apnea in this population.

Patients with Down syndrome also have alterations in the paranasal sinuses,[9] abnormalities of serum immunoglobulins,[10] and ciliary dyskinesia,[11] which contribute to the high incidence of chronic sinusitis.

In addition, these patients have many comorbidities that must be considered by the surgeon and anesthesiologist:

- Congenital heart disease
- Pulmonary hypertension
- Gastroesophageal reflux disease (GERD)
- Subglottic stenosis
- Cervical instability.

As care for patients with Down syndrome has been deinstitutionalized in recent decades, and as more of these children are cared for by their parents, integration into schools and social acceptance of these patients has grown. Because of this, more resources have been made available to help these children integrate into society and lead fulfilled, productive, and independent lives. The role of the otolaryngologist in these patients' lives can be significant. Although most needed in childhood, the otolaryngologist plays a role throughout the life of the patient with Down syndrome (**Fig. 1**).

PRENATAL FINDINGS IN DOWN SYNDROME

On rare occasion, the otolaryngologist may be consulted because of a lack of nasal bones as seen on prenatal ultrasound. A total of approximately 49,000 fetuses from

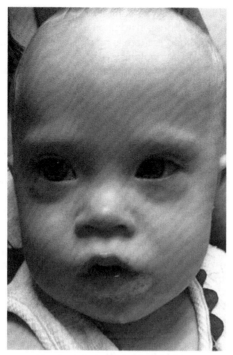

Fig. 1. Child with Down syndrome with characteristic facies.

several studies yields a prevalence of nasal bone absence of 65% in trisomy 21 and 1% to 3% in euploid fetuses.[12] If nasal bone evaluation is to be used in screening for Down syndrome, it is important to have sonographers who are trained to perform such evaluations. Differences in studies have ranged from a reported rate of 16.7% for absent nasal bones in fetuses with trisomy 21 evaluated by sonographers without training or quality assurance,[13] to 70% prevalence in studies in which sonographers were appropriately trained.

In the first trimester, the purpose of an ultrasound evaluation of the nasal bones is to recognize whether the nasal bones are present or absent.[14] Ultrasound assessment of nasal bones, in addition to several other ultrasound markers, can increase the performance of first-trimester screening tests to greater than 90% for a fixed false-positive rate of 5%.[15]

In the second trimester, the screening focuses on nasal bone length, with hypoplastic nasal bones being the marker for Down syndrome. Hypoplastic nasal bones are defined as absent or shorter than 2.5 mm.[16] It has been shown that using sonographic markers of prenasal thickness, nasal bone length, and nuchal skin fold increased the detection of Down syndrome in the second trimester by 19% to 23% compared with serum markers alone.[17] This rate of 93% detection for a fixed false-positive rate of 5% is comparable with first-trimester screening protocols.[17] Although absent nasal bones are an important additional finding in prenatal screening, the significance of an isolated finding of absent nasal bones is less clear. One study showed that, in 14 patients with absent nasal bones, only 6 had Down syndrome and 8 had a normal karyotype.[18] In this study, 6 of 6, 100% of fetuses with the isolated finding of absent nasal bones had normal karyotypes; however, 6 of 8 (75%) of the patients who had absent nasal bones in addition to other abnormal ultrasound findings did have Down syndrome. Although there is no role for otolaryngologic intervention at this time, it is helpful for otolaryngologists to be familiar with this screening tool, because they may be consulted for an opinion or assessment.

THE EAR IN DOWN SYNDROME

The ears of the patient with Down syndrome are likely the reason for the first encounter with the otolaryngologist. Patients with Down syndrome have a range of otologic problems including stenotic ear canals, increased incidence of secretory otitis media, chronic ear disease, and secondary hearing loss, as well as hearing loss caused by ossicular abnormalities and inner ear dysplasia. In early life, it has been estimated that 40% to 50% of newborns with Down syndrome have stenotic ear canals.[19] These factors may make it difficult for the pediatrician to adequately examine the ear by otoscopic examination.

PEARLS and PITFALLS: These narrowed canals predispose the patient with Down syndrome to cerumen impaction, and the cerumen combined with the stenotic canal makes it difficult to adequately examine the ear. Further, it has been observed that patients with stenotic ear canals had a markedly increased incidence of associated middle ear effusions.[19] It is recommended that children with Down syndrome establish care with an otolaryngologist early in life, because the patient will frequently require microscopic examinations and cerumen disimpaction of the canals under microscopy. It is also recommended that those with canal stenosis continue to follow up every 3 months with the otolaryngologist for evaluation of the middle ear space, to ensure that there is no cerumen impaction, and to monitor for middle ear fluid and infection (Fig. 2).

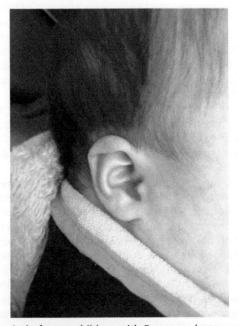

Fig. 2. Folded helix typical of many children with Down syndrome.

Further research is needed on the natural progression of canal stenosis; however, the experience reported by Cincinnati Children's Hospital is that most children with stenotic canals grow with age, and by years 2 or 3 this canal is no longer an obstacle to accurate examination.[20] Each patient should be followed regularly by an otolaryngologist until it is clear that the patients are of appropriate age and size so that they are at low risk of serous otitis media and can be easily examined.

Cause of Ear Problems in Children with Down Syndrome

The high prevalence of serous otitis media in children with Down syndrome has been well documented in the academic literature.[21,22] Several causal factors explain this increased incidence of ear disease:

- Children with Down syndrome have an increased number of upper respiratory infections, possibly caused by the reduction of both T and B lymphocyte function,[10,23] impaired body response to specific pathogens, and defective neutrophil chemotaxis.[24]
- Patients with Down syndrome also have midface anatomy that predisposes them to chronic ear disease. The midface hypoplasia seen in many patients with Down syndrome involves the nasopharynx and the eustachian tube openings.
- A study on the radiographic features of patients with Down syndrome showed that the bony confines of the nasopharynx were smaller in children with Down syndrome, and therefore the normal-sized soft tissue of the nasopharynx can only occupy this space at the expense of the airway.[25] This decrease in postnasal space may cause even small to medium-sized adenoids to give rise to eustachian tube dysfunction.
- It has also been shown that the eustachian tubes in these patients are extremely small, and collapsed in several portions.[6] A histopathologic study of eustachian tubes in patients with Down syndrome compared with controls showed that the cartilage cell density in individuals with Down syndrome was decreased at all ages, predisposing the canal to collapse.[26] Further, it has been hypothesized that the generalized hypotonia of these patients can lead to decreased function of the tensor veli palatini muscle of the palate, which is responsible for opening the eustachian tube.[19] These factors combine to cause collapse of the eustachian tube. This collapse can cause negative pressure in the middle ear space and result in chronic otitis media and fluid accumulation.
- In addition to the eustachian tube dysfunction, there may be factors within the middle ear that contribute to disease. In a study of otitis media, Ts65Dn mice, which share many phenotypic characteristics of human Down syndrome, were used as a model for human Down syndrome.[27] When examined, 11 of 15 of the Ts65Dn mice had middle ear effusions, compared with only 2 of 11 of the wild-type mice. On histopathologic examination, the Ts65Dn mice had thickened mucosa and goblet cells were distributed with higher density in the epithelium of the middle ear cavity. Also, bacteria of pathogenic importance to humans were identified in these mice. If these characteristics are also present in the child with Down syndrome, these children are likely to have recurring ear infections.

The causal conditions of secretory otitis media are many, and the impact on the hearing of a child with Down syndrome can be profound. In one study, 90% of children had at least a mild-moderate hearing loss. Despite the high point prevalence of hearing loss in this sample group, only a small percentage of parents (15.2%) reported a positive history of hearing loss.[28]

Hearing Loss in Down Syndrome

It has been documented that hearing loss in children with Down syndrome is more frequent than in healthy children.[29] In studies that conducted audio screening on randomly selected children with Down syndrome, 50% to 90% of children with Down syndrome had a hearing impairment.[21,28,30,31] Hearing impairment may be masked in patients with intellectual impairment, because speech delays, and lack of response to verbal cues, may be attributed to mental retardation.

> PEARLS and PITFALLS: *It is particularly important for the otolaryngologist to monitor these patients because they are especially susceptible to otitis media and its resulting conductive hearing loss.*

Detection of this loss is critical, because the detrimental effects of hearing loss on language development are thought to be greater for children with learning disabilities compared with children without mental retardation.[32,33] The American Academy of Pediatrics Committee on Genetic and the Down Syndrome Interest Group Guideline recommends audiologic testing at birth, then every 6 months up to age 3 years, with annual testing after 3 years of age, or when ear-specific pure tone audiometry may be obtained (**Fig. 3**).[34,35]

> PEARLS and PITFALLS: *It is recommended that all children with Down syndrome have routine audiologic screening.*

Audiologic Evaluation for Children with Down Syndrome

The initial audiologic evaluation is done by auditory brainstem response (ABR) or otoacoustic emissions (OAE). As the patient grows older, the preferred method of audiologic testing is debated.

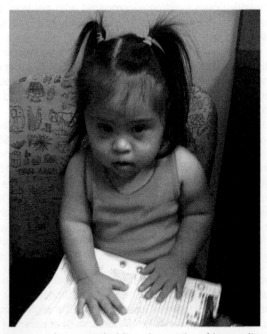

Fig. 3. Child with Down syndrome sits holding the results of her audiogram.

The evaluation of hearing by behavioral audiometry in young patients is frequently challenging, and is made more difficult in patients who are intellectually challenged. The patient with Down syndrome may have a limited voluntary response during testing, because of a lack of attention and poor psychomotor skills. Further, this type of sound-field testing does not differentiate between ears, because it evaluates both ears together, so a unilateral hearing loss can be missed.

It was shown in a Chinese study that combined objective testing using tympanometry and transitory evoked otoacoustic emission (TEOAE) is a feasible protocol for screening school-aged children with Down syndrome.[28] The TEOAE is able to detect mild hearing loss, but may be inaccurate in the presence of middle ear fluid. The tympanometry and pneumatic otoscopy by the otolaryngologist compliments the examination to screen for hearing loss. However, the TEOAE is costly, limiting accessibility to some patients. Because of cost restrictions, most patients with Down syndrome go for biannual testing using behavioral audiometry, which should be performed by an audiologist who is experienced in behavioral testing and familiar with patients with Down syndrome.

CONDUCTIVE LOSS CAUSED BY EFFUSION OR OTITIS MEDIA
Tympanostomy in Patients with Down Syndrome

The benefits of PE tubes in patients with Down syndrome has been debated during the past decade. The clinical efficacy of tympanostomy tubes has been well established for OME in the general population, with reports that tympanostomy tubes decrease the duration of middle ear effusion compared with no surgical intervention.[36] However, in the patient with Down syndrome, results have been varied.

One study examined the short-term effects of PE tubes, measured by pure tone audiometry, 6 to 9 weeks after tube placement.[37] This study found improved hearing in only 60% of patients with Down syndrome, compared with 91% improvement in the control group. In this study, all patients were older than 6 years (mean age 8.1 years), and none had had PE tubes placed in the past. In the Down syndrome population, which is particularly vulnerable to early onset and prolonged duration of secretary otitis media, this delay of treatment could be the cause of failure, rather than the treatment itself.

A study in Japan also showed poor outcomes in children with Down syndrome, and a high complication rate.[38] This study found that few (21.4%) children were cured of OME by age 7 years, after the initial set of PE tubes was placed, whereas nearly 88% of controls were cured in this same time frame. Reviewing this study revealed faults that do not necessarily indicate treatment failure:

- The mean age of these children was 5.4 years, which may be past the critical point in intervening in the Down syndrome population.
- The important finding in this study was that most children with Down syndrome had recurrent OME after extrusion of tubes. In normal controls, the incidence of OME is reported to peak in infancy and decline rapidly after the age of 6 years, when the immune system and eustachian tube have reached maturity.[39] However, it has been shown that OME persists for a longer period in children with Down syndrome,[40] and that the canal stenosis, and the highly viscous nature of the mucous expressed, often require further insertion of tympanostomy tubes.[41] The population studied by Iino and colleagues[38] may have had greater success had tubes been reinserted in all patients.
- There was a high rate of complications in this study in the patients with Down syndrome compared with controls. Sequelae of OME were found in 15 of 50 of the ears in the Down syndrome group including 4 cholesteatomas, 9 permanent perforations, and 2 atelactatic tympanic membranes. This complication rate has

not been reported in other studies; however, it is important to consider when deciding between conservative management and surgical intervention.

Special Considerations in Surgical Management of the Child with Down Syndrome

It is clear from the aforementioned literature that the patient with Down syndrome cannot be treated with the same timeline and same algorithms that are used for the nonsyndromic child. If surgical management is the chosen path, results must be closely monitored, and the surgeon must be aggressive with reintervention. This has been shown by a study at the Cincinnati Children's Hospital[42]:

- Children with Down syndrome were enrolled before the age of 2 years
- The children were followed by an otolaryngologist every 3 to 6 months, depending on the degree of canal stenosis present
- All children were treated for chronic ear infections and middle ear effusions by placement of PE tubes, and replacement tubes as needed
- At the end of the study 2 years later, 93% of the patients had normal hearing
- The children with Down syndrome with the PE tubes in place had a 3.6 times higher chance of having normal hearing compared with the audiograms of children with Down syndrome who presented at a similar age as the children finishing the study, but had not had aggressive management of OME and did not have PE tubes in place.

Also reinforcing this concept is a study on receptive and expressive language in adolescents with Down syndrome.[43] In this study:

- Adolescents who had tympanostomy tubes placed when they were children showed significantly higher language scores than did the group of patients who had more than 3 known infections as a child, but never had tubes placed
- Effects of temporary hearing loss associated with otitis media may play an important role in the language deficits so commonly seen in individuals with Down syndrome
- Effects of the hearing loss extend far beyond the time course of the disease itself.

Surgical intervention by placement of PE tubes can be an effective strategy in the management of patients with Down syndrome with OME refractory to medical therapy. However, the otolaryngologist must counsel the parents of the patient about the possible increased risks in these patients, including cholesteatoma, persistent perforation, and atelectatic tympanic membranes.

The study by Iino and colleagues[38,40] had a nearly 30% complication rate, which they attribute in part to the eardrums of children with Down syndrome being thin, which can be seen while applying force to the drum with the pneumatic otoscope or while performing myringotomy.[39] They state that a thin eardrum lacks a lamina propria, which lack blood vessels and collagen fibers and are susceptible to permanent perforation. Parents must be prepared for the possibility that the patient may have persistent otorrhea after tube placement.[39] Also, parents must understand that the treatment of OME in the child with Down syndrome may differ from the treatment they may be familiar with or have experienced through other children. They should know that the PE tubes may be placed earlier in the child's life, and should expect that the child may need multiple set of tubes throughout childhood, even into adulthood. They should be counseled that reinsertion of tubes is a continuation of treatment, rather than failure of the original attempt. Parents should be counseled on the importance of follow-up with the audiologist and the otolaryngologist, and the need for aggressive intervention and reintervention in order for the procedure to be successful at preventing hearing loss.

CONDUCTIVE LOSS CAUSED BY MASTOID OR OSSICULAR CHAIN ABNORMALITIES

In addition to middle ear effusions, a component of conductive loss may be caused by abnormalities of the mastoid, or abnormality of the ossicular chain. A study reviewed neuroimaging of 59 patients with Down syndrome and found nonaeration or underaeration of mastoids in most (74%) cases.[44] This finding agrees with a previous study, showing 63% of the mastoids examined on lateral cervical spine films with sclerosis and poor aeration.[45] Whether this increase in density is caused by a mastoid infection that occurred during maximum growth years or a congenital component is yet to be determined. A study examining 107 patients with Down syndrome found that only 60% of the conductive hearing loss could be explained by middle ear effusions or tympanic membrane perforations. This finding prompted the investigators to examine the temporal bones of 5 Down syndrome cadavers, as well as document operating room findings during middle ear surgery in these patients. Ossicular abnormalities were attributed to chronic disease, including erosion of the long process of the incus, of the manubrium of the malleus, and of the superstructure of the stapes. Some findings were also attributed to congenital deformities, including malformation of the stapes and dehiscence of the facial nerve.[46] These findings should be considered in children who have a persistent conductive hearing loss despite maximal management of middle ear effusion.

The increased incidence of chronic ear disease in patients with Down syndrome predisposes them to cholesteatoma and erosion of the ossicular chain. Although the 1979 study by Balkany and colleagues[46] found little improvement in conductive hearing loss in patients with Down syndrome who underwent reconstructive surgery for ossicular chain abnormalities, a more recent study by O'Malley and colleagues[47] in 2007 gives more promising results. This study is the largest to date on ear surgery for chronic conditions, including 21 patients with Down syndrome, among 22 other patients with congenital syndromes. This study showed that such patients, including those with Down syndrome, can successfully eradicate disease with creation of a safe, dry ear, and that ossicular chain reconstruction techniques significantly improved hearing in this population.[47] Parents should be counseled that resolution of disease may require several operations. In the this study, 64% of ears were managed with a single surgery, and 89% of ears were controlled with 2 surgeries or fewer. Similarly, parents should also be counseled that canal wall preservation techniques may not be appropriate for this population. In patients with Down syndrome with cholesteatoma in this study, 70% of patients required a canal wall down study, and 89% of patients required a canal wall down procedure in a study of 9 patients with Down syndrome.[48] These procedures have been successful in eradication of disease in this population, but parents should be counseled appropriately about the likelihood of reoperation and the difficulty of using canal wall sparing procedures.

MIXED AND SENSORINEURAL HEARING LOSS IN CHILDREN WITH DOWN SYNDROME

In addition to the conductive hearing loss caused by otitis media and middle ear effusion, children with Down syndrome also have higher rates of mixed hearing loss and sensorineural hearing loss compared with other children. It is difficult to determine what percentage of this is caused by chronic middle ear disease and osteoid deposition in the fundus of the internal auditory canal and the region of the spiral tract, through which nerve bundles cross from the inner ear to the internal auditory canal.

The true incidence of sensorineural hearing loss in children with Down syndrome will be determined as future studies evaluate hearing in children who have been aided by early and aggressive care of their middle ear disease. Although the exact figure of sensorineural hearing loss is difficult to determine, studies evaluating hearing in patients with Down syndrome have found it to be 4% to 9%.[21,30] Several studies have examined inner ear anomalies that may contribute to hearing loss. One study found them to have uniformly small inner ear structures compared with controls, including hypoplastic cochlea, critically smaller cochlear nerve canal, narrowed internal auditory canal, hypoplastic lateral semicircular canal with a small bony island, and hypoplastic vestibules.[43]

Options to Enhance Hearing of Patients with Down Syndrome

Bone-anchored hearing aid

Early reports on other options to enhance the hearing of patients with Down syndrome are promising. The bone-anchored hearing aid (BAHA) has been successfully used in patients with Down syndrome who failed conventional hearing aids and ventilation tubes. A review of BAHA centers in Ireland and the United Kingdom showed that 18 of 81 BAHA centers are performing surgery on patients with Down syndrome.[49] Of the 43 patients with Down syndrome who were implanted, all but 1 wore the BAHA on a daily basis, which indicates a high level of patient satisfaction.

A survey on perceived patient and parent/caregiver satisfaction was completed by the centers, and showed that 27 of 28 were very pleased or pleased with the results. Similarly, a study surveying 15 patients with BAHA found all 15 using the BAHA regularly, with audiologic benefit.[50]

To evaluate the overall benefit of the BAHA, the Glasgow Children's Benefit Inventory was used, which evaluates emotion, physical health, learning, and vitality. The results of this study showed a significant benefit in all categories in children with Down syndrome.

Complications in the first study were 50%, which is significantly higher than the previously reported 9% to 16% in nonsyndromic children and 32% in adults. The complication rate in the second study was 20%. In both, the most common complications were soft tissue problems, including excessive healing of the graft site with hypertrophy of soft tissues, graft infection, and skin reaction. All were resolved within a short time, usually within 2 months. The increase in soft tissue complications in patients with Down syndrome may be attributed to patients with learning difficulties having a tendency to interfere with the area, leading to disturbances of the dressing, sutures, and possible graft failure. A solution to this was proposed, in which, following BAHA abutment, a perforated thermoplastic cage is formed over the surgical site and sutured into place. The empirical evidence within this practice has shown this to be effective.[51]

Cochlear implants

Cochlear implants were originally not recommended for patients with additional disabilities beyond hearing loss. However, with a growing body of knowledge and good results, inclusion criteria are expanding and there are now increasing numbers of such candidates, including patients with Down syndrome.

A study published in 2010 reported that at least 4 patients with Down syndrome had received cochlear implants in the United Kingdom and Ireland.[52] In all cases, the deafness was congenital, and all 4 of the patients had middle ear disease before surgery, with 2 patients requiring PE tubes. However, all of the patients were treated before surgery and none of the cases had any complications associated with otitis media.

Despite the previous discussion of mastoid underaeration and opacification, inner ear dysplasia, shortened cochlear lengths, and dehiscent facial nerve, none of the patients implanted had any of these findings and none had intraoperative difficulties.

The outcomes for these 4 implanted patients have been modest gains in auditory performance, with the eldest child, who has had the implant the longest, showing the most improvement. As more patients with Down syndrome become candidates for cochlear implants, patients and families must be counseled about expectations. There are abnormalities in the temporal bone of a child with Down syndrome that may increase the risk of complications. Even in technically successful implantation, the outcomes may not be as good as in children without additional disabilities, because learning and communication difficulties may prolong the rehabilitation. However, these patients do show improvement, and future patients with Down syndrome with profound sensorineural hearing loss may be referred for assessment at cochlear implant programs.

Sound-field amplification and speech/language intervention
In addition to surgical options, initial studies using sound-field amplification and speech/language intervention have shown excellent results.

A pilot study tested an aggressive multidisciplinary model consisting of amplification technology and speech/language intervention that emphasizes auditory-verbal therapy, as well as aggressive medical and surgical management of ear disorders.[53] This program was initiated in children with Down syndrome less than 1 year old. The findings in these 6 children enrolled in the program were that the children in the intervention group had developed age-appropriate early language skills, with no apparent gap between their receptive and oral expressive language abilities. A group of children with Down syndrome of the same age who did not have the intervention were used as comparison, and the no-intervention group had generalized language delays with a noticeable gap between receptive understanding and oral expressive language.

Another study examined the benefits of sound-field amplification in 4 children with Down syndrome in the classroom setting.[54] The study found that that participant's speech perception significantly improved when the FM sound-field amplification was being used. The sound-field amplifier is recommended rather than a traditional hearing aid in this population, because the sound-field amplifier selectively amplifies the teacher's voice, which improves the signal/noise ratio, whereas the hearing aid increases all sounds equally, including background noise that can be distracting. In the patients with Down syndrome, who are prone to fluctuating conductive hearing loss, the effects of poor classroom acoustics are significant.

As more of these children with Down syndrome are mainstreamed and placed in public schools, additional support is needed to achieve full potential. More outcomes research is needed, but sound-field amplifiers have the potential to improve classroom performance.

OBSTRUCTIVE SLEEP APNEA AND SLEEP DISORDERED BREATHING

Although OSAS is seen in only 0.7% to 2.0% of the general pediatric population,[55,56] the prevalence in pediatric patients with Down syndrome has been estimated at 77% to 80%.[57,58] Children with Down syndrome have many predisposing factors of OSAS:

- Midfacial and mandibular hypoplasia[59] glossoptosis
- An abnormally small upper airway with superficially positioned tonsils and relative tonsillar and adenoidal encroachment[8]
- Increased secretions

- Increased incidence of lower respiratory tract anomalies
- Obesity and generalized hypotonia with resultant collapse of the airway during inspiration.

Children with OSAS have a worsened trend in word reading speed, visual attention, and verbal fluency.[60] OSAS has been shown to result in neurodevelopmental problems such as daytime somnolence, behavioral disturbances, school failure, and developmental delay.[61] Obstructive sleep apnea can cause pulmonary hypertension resulting in cor pulmonale and congestive heart failure secondary to the chronic, intermittent hypoxemia and respiratory acidosis during sleep.[62] Although we know of no published studies specifically examining these effects of neurodevelopment and learning on children with Down syndrome, it is logical to expect that this population, already predisposed to learning delay and difficulty in school, would be significantly impaired by the effects of sleep apnea. Similarly, children with Down syndrome are predisposed to congenital cardiac anomalies and are more likely to have pulmonary hypertension than are nonsyndromic children with the same cardiac anomalies.[63] Again, this may be exacerbated or worsened by OSAS (**Fig. 4**).

PEARLS and PITFALLS: Children with Down syndrome have many predisposing factors of OSAS.

Diagnosing Obstructive Sleep Apnea in Children with Down Syndrome

The diagnosis of OSAS should come from an overnight polysomnography whenever possible. A study examined 53 patients with Down syndrome for OSAS by nap study and, of those, 16 patients had both a nap polysomnography and an overnight polysomnography.[53] All 16 (100%) had abnormal overnight polysomnograms, but the nap study was less sensitive in detecting OSAS, with only 12 (75%) of these patients

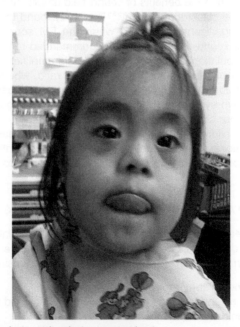

Fig. 4. Midface hypoplasia with relative macroglossia.

having abnormal nap studies. The degrees of hypoventilation and desaturations were significantly higher in the overnight studies, and thus the nap studies, under estimated abnormalities.

Snoring in sleep apnea diagnosis

The diagnosis of sleep apnea is not limited to the children with Down syndrome who snore, although those who do snore have a high likelihood of having a positive sleep study. In a retrospective review of patients with Down syndrome who were referred for polysomnography because of snoring, 97% of these snoring patients had a positive sleep study.[64] The child with Down syndrome who is not reported to snore is still at significant risk for sleep apnea and should be evaluated.

Parental reporting of sleep apnea

It may be difficult for a parent to tell whether a child is suffering from sleep apnea, because the most severe apneic events often happen during rapid eye movement (REM) sleep, late at night, when the parents are also asleep. In the child with Down syndrome, the parents may assume that their child's irregular breathing at night is normal for a child with Down syndrome, which is a frequently expressed comment.[58] Parental reports are not reliable in ruling out sleep apnea.

A study showed that 11 of 35 (31%) of parents of children with Down syndrome reported that their children had sleep problems, but these parents were correct about a sleep abnormality in only about 4 of 11 (36%) cases. The other 7 of 11 (64%) had normal polysomnograms. Of the 24 of 35 (69%) parents who reported no sleep problems, 13 of 24 (54%) of the children had abnormal polysomnograms, and did have obstructive sleep apnea.[58]

In another study, 19 of 49 children (39%) had histories that suggested OSAS. Polysomnograms were abnormal in all 19 (100%) of the patients with a positive history. However, 18 of 30 (60%) of the children with negative histories also had abnormal polysomnograms.

Because of the unreliability of parental reporting, the high prevalence of OSAS in this population, and the negative effects of sleep apnea, it is recommended that all children with Down syndrome between the ages of 3 and 4 years go for objective testing using full overnight polysomnography for a baseline study.[58]

Risk Factors for OSAS

Because of the possibility of health problems associated with OSAS in a population already at higher health risk, learning about the cause of the disease is important.

One established risk factor for obstructive sleep apnea (OSA) in adults and children in the general population is high body mass index (BMI), and weight reduction is often effective at decreasing the effects of sleep apnea.[65] However, the correlation between BMI and OSAS in the patient with Down syndrome is not so clear.

- A study surveyed consecutively encountered, nonselected patients with Down syndrome. Seventy-nine percent of them had OSAS, and higher BMI was significantly associated with a higher apnea index and lower arterial oxygen saturation (Sao_2) level.[66]
- A study in 2010 compared age-matched children with Down syndrome with OSA and without OSA based on polysomnogram results.[67] The mean BMI z-score was statistically significantly different between OSA and non-OSA groups, with the OSAS group having a BMI z-score of 2.09 and the non–sleep apnea group a BMI z-score of 1.4. The BMI z-score, also called BMI standard deviation score, are measures of relative weight adjusted for the child's age and sex.[68] However, there

were some patients in this review who had an extremely high BMI who had a normal sleep study, and several patients with a low BMI did have OSAS.

- Similarly, in the study by Fitzgerald and colleagues[64] in 2007, 91% of the study subjects were not obese, but 97% had OSA and 50% of those had severe OSA.

Based on these results, OSAS is likely a multifactorial disease with several contributing factors in these patients. However, BMI is a modifiable risk factor, and the results of the studies discussed earlier suggest that weight reduction may show some benefit in the management of OSA in children with Down syndrome (**Fig. 5**).

PEARLS and PITFALLS: A preoperative polysomnogram is now recommended in patients with Down syndrome before tonsillectomy and/or adenoidecomty.[71]

Tonsil and Adenoid Surgery in the Child with Down Syndrome

Before entertaining tonsil and adenoid surgery in the Down syndrome population, it is now recommended that a preoperative polysomnography is obtained.[69] For children who are diagnosed with OSAS after a sleep study, the initial surgical treatment of OSAS is tonsillectomy and adenoidectomy,[70] including for children with Down syndrome. The efficacy of tonsillectomy and adenoidectomy in curing sleep apnea in patients with Down syndrome is generally accepted to be lower, with 30% to 50% of patients with Down syndrome requiring CPAP support, further surgery, or tracheostomy at a later date.[8,71] A recently published article confirms this, giving exact data on preoperative and postoperative polysomnograms in both children with Down syndrome and nonsyndromic children who served as age-matched and BMI-matched controls.[72]

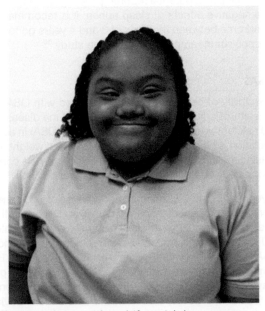

Fig. 5. Child with Down syndrome with multifactorial sleep apnea.

- In the Down syndrome group, the Apnea Hypopnea Index (AHI) showed improvement after surgery, but was not as significant as the improvement in the control group.
- The REM-AHI and lowest Sao_2 did not show significant change in the children with Down syndrome, whereas all respiratory parameters improved in the control children.
- None of the nonsyndromic children required CPAP or further surgery after tonsillectomy and adenoidectomy, despite having increased BMI (average 27.6). Seventy-three percent of the children with Down syndrome went on to require CPAP, biphasic positive airway pressure, and supplemental oxygen for persistent OSA after tonsillectomy and adenoidectomy.

This cure rate is lower than the rate previously cited, in which 48% of patients with Down syndrome had a persistently increased AHI after tonsillectomy and adenoidectomy.[73] The variability between these 2 outcomes is likely caused by patient comorbidities, because it has been shown that patients with multiple comorbidities have poorer outcomes in curing OSA.[74]

Managing outcome expectations of tonsillectomy and adenoidectomy for OSA
Although the success rates of tonsillectomy and adenoidectomy in curing sleep apnea in children with Down syndrome is different from the rates in nonsyndromic children, the procedure may still be recommended if the parents are given appropriate information about expectations and can give informed consent.

> PEARLS and PITFALLS: *It is important to ensure that parents expect tonsillectomy and adenoidectomy to provide an improvement in symptoms in the patient with Down syndrome, rather than a complete cure.*

In the aforementioned study by Shete and colleagues,[72] all patients showed some improvement in AHI after tonsillectomy and adenoidectomy. Although we know of no exact data, this improvement in AHI and partial relief of obstruction may decrease the need for CPAP or oxygen. Although the patient may still require supplemental breathing support at night, the setting on the CPAP may be decreased, resulting in greater patient comfort. CPAP compliance is low in normal adults,[75] and it is even more difficult for children with a developmental disability, who do not understand the disease or the treatment, to be fully compliant. Therefore, a likelihood of reducing dependence on CPAP, and/or a 25% to 50% chance of being weaned completely from a nighttime breathing apparatus, may make the surgery a good option for many patients with Down syndrome.

Risks of Tonsillectomy and Adenoidectomy in the Child with Down Syndrome

In addition to managing parental expectations about the success of tonsillectomy and adenoidectomy, parents also need to be counseled on the risks. A questionnaire survey of 74 parents of children with Down syndrome was conducted and found that 2 of 74 patients developed transient velopharyngeal insufficiency (VPI), and an additional 2 of 74 patients reported permanent hypernasal speech after adenotonsillectomy.[76]

Although it is difficult to extrapolate from this to determine the frequency with which VPI and hypernasality occur in patients with Down syndrome after tonsillectomy and adenoidectomy, it is presumably significantly higher than the 1:2000 to 1:3000 rate of complications seen in the general population.[77,78]

When given complete evaluation, patients who reported complications were found to have both structural and functional causes of hypernasality:

- Structural causes of hypernasality included a high arched and short soft palate
- The functional component included hypotonia, slowed motor learning, and oral motor developmental delay.

From this information, it can be assumed that all patients with Down syndrome are at higher risk of developing VPI or hypernasality after surgery, because the characteristics listed earlier are common to patients with Down syndrome.

A different study reviewed postoperative complications in children with Down syndrome compared with controls, and found a higher incidence of complications in the Down syndrome group after adenotonsillectomy[79]:

- Increased hospital stay
- Fivefold increase in respiratory complications requiring intervention
- Increased duration until adequate oral intake.

It is therefore recommended that all patients with Down syndrome be admitted to the hospital after adenotonsillectomy for observation.[79] Parents should be counseled on the risks before surgery, and special precautions and preparations should be made on a case-by-case basis, based on the child's condition and comorbidities.

PEARLS and PITFALLS: It is recommended that all patients with Down syndrome be admitted to the hospital after surgery for observation and monitoring.[79]

Managing Refractory Obstructive Sleep Apnea in the Child with Down Syndrome

Most patients who have persistent OSAS after tonsillectomy can be treated with CPAP. CPAP can be an effective therapy, but the therapeutic benefit of CPAP is limited by poor patient compliance, especially in the pediatric population. For this reason, patients often prefer a surgical option if one is available. The next step in surgical treatment, after tonsillectomy and adenoidectomy, is more complex.

Patients with Down syndrome have anatomy that predisposes them to multilevel airway collapse, and preoperative planning must identify the level responsible for collapse as well as the severity. Standard work-up has included history and physical examination, including flexible nasopharyngoscopy to the level of the larynx.

Sleep nasoendoscopy

Sleep nasoendoscopy has been used to determine sites of airway obstruction. In this procedure, the child is put in a supine position and administered light sedation with spontaneous respirations. Flexible endoscopy is performed and the airways are evaluated and recorded.[80] However, this technique is flawed, because the entire airway cannot be seen at one time, so the effects of sequential obstruction cannot be evaluated (ie, how one level of obstruction affects a second level).

Cine magnetic resonance imaging

Recently, cine magnetic resonance imaging (MRI) has been used with good results to assist in planning additional surgical intervention.[71,81] Cine MRI was originally used by neurosurgeons to evaluate cerebrospinal fluid flow in real time. Now it is being used in some institutions to assess sleep apnea. In the case of sleep apnea, the patient is placed supine on the table, sleep is induced by sleep deprivation, spontaneous sleep, or sedation. The evaluation is most accurate if imaging takes place when the patient is snoring or having apneic events during spontaneous respirations. The cine MRI obtains multiple sagittal and axial images in real time, creating a dynamic, three-dimensional video of the airway collapse. This view can appreciate multiple levels of collapse, and it has also been noted that adenoid enlargement and nasopharyngeal obstruction are more prominent on cine MRI.[80]

Subsequent aggressive surgical treatment

Although many patients may go on to need further surgery for OSAS, there are no data to support more aggressive surgery initially. A study examined patients with Down syndrome who underwent tonsillectomy and adenoidectomy, and patients with Down syndrome who underwent tonsillectomy and adenoidectomy plus lateral pharyngoplasty as initial therapy for OSAS. There was no significant difference between the groups, with 48% in the tonsillectomy and adenoidectomy–only group having persistently abnormal AHI after surgery, and 63% in the tonsillectomy and adenoidectomy plus lateral pharyngoplasty group having abnormal AHI after surgery.[70] Therefore, it is recommended that tonsillectomy and adenoidectomy alone be the initial surgical treatment, and the patient may return for subsequent treatment if this procedure is not curative.

Genioglossus advancement and radiofrequency ablation

Data were recently published on combined genioglossus advancement and radiofrequency ablation of the tongue base in pediatric patients with OSAS refractory to tonsillectomy and adenoidectomy. In this study, 61% of the patients had Down syndrome.[82] Successful outcome was achieved in 12 of 19 patients with Down syndrome, resulting in AHI of less than 5, maintaining an oxygen saturation of greater than 90% throughout the night, and end tidal CO_2 of more than 50 mm Hg for less than 10% of the total sleep time. The findings of this study support treatment of refractory OSA with genioglossus advancement and radiofrequency ablation in the Down syndrome population. Although this report is promising, further research is needed supporting and validating other methods of treating refractory OSA with multilevel obstruction.

RHINITIS AND SINUSITIS IN THE PATIENT WITH DOWN SYNDROME

The patient with Down syndrome is predisposed to chronic nasal drainage, nasal obstruction, and sinusitis caused by the narrowing of the nose and nasal sinuses. One study of patients with Down syndrome found that 17.6% of children with Down syndrome were reported to have a continually runny nose.[37] The narrowing of the nasopharynx leads normal growth of adenoid tissue to obstruct the airway, predisposing patients to nasal congestion and subsequent infection. In addition, several studies have shown abnormalities in the immunoglobulin (Ig) levels in Down syndrome,[10,23,83] with IgG4 subclass deficiency the most common finding in patients with recurrent infection.[84] A review of immunologic features of Down syndrome describes that, although the primary immune defect seems to be greatest in the cellular compartment, even the humoral immunity in subjects with Down syndrome undergoes a precocious aging.[24] An anatomically small and obstructed nasopharynx combined with decreased immunity predisposes the patient with Down syndrome to chronic rhinorrhea and sinusitis.

Medical Treatment of Rhinitis and Sinusitis in the Child with Down Syndrome

Treatment of this nasal drainage is similar to treatment in the general population, with nasal irrigation, nasal steroids, antihistamines, decongestants, and antibiotics as needed. One study treated 25 children with Down syndrome empirically with low-dose ampicillin daily, from the onset of symptoms until May. This treatment gave an excellent response, as reported by parents.[8]

Surgical Treatment of Rhinitis and Sinusitis in the Child with Down Syndrome

In patients whose sinusitis and rhinitis are not aided by medical management, surgical intervention may be warranted. Flexible nasopharyngoscopy should be preformed to look for adenoid hypertrophy, which may be obstructing the choanae. This nasopharyngoscopy should be done even if the patient has already had an adenoidectomy, because regrowth of adenoid tissue is more common in the patient with Down syndrome compared with the general population.[80] If the patient does have obstructing adenoid tissue, it is important to know that adenoidectomy is less effective in treating nasal and middle ear syndromes in children with Down syndrome compared with controls.

One study examined adenoidectomy in children with Down syndrome compared with controls, and the efficacy in treatment of nasal obstruction, snoring, mouth breathing, and middle ear disease. The findings were that, although some of the patients with Down syndrome improved, the percentage of patients who were symptom free after adenoidectomy was significantly lower than in the control group with nearly every symptom. As with all surgical interventions, parents should be counseled before surgery and given expectations for improvement, not necessarily a cure. The physical examination and nasal endoscopy should assess septal deviation, as well as turbinate hypertrophy that may be amenable to surgical correction. If the patient continues to have persistent sinusitis despite maximal medical therapy, then a computed tomography scan of the sinuses is recommend. Based on the results, functional endoscopic sinus surgery may be warranted.

Rapid Maxillary Expansion

A new method of treating nasal obstruction is currently being explored; rapid maxillary expansion (RME) has been used to augment nasal volume and reduce ear, nose, and throat infections. RME is an orthodontic procedure used to correct a narrow transverse maxillary diameter.

The 2 maxillary bones are separated at the midpalatal structure using an intraoral screw mechanism. This separation leads to a widening of the perimeter of the arch. Although the major effect is noticed clinically in the area of dentition, the transverse enlargement of the apical bone also affects nasal width. These changes usually result in altered nasal airway flow, with consequently improved nasal ventilation.[85]

In this study, 13 patients with Down syndrome used the intraoral maxillary expansion device and 10 patients with Down syndrome did not. The results showed a significant increase in the total nasal volume, which persisted 5 months after removal of the device.[86] The study further reported a significantly lower incidence of acute otitis media, adenoiditis, and tonsillitis in the RME group, as well as improved severity of snoring, mouth breathing, restlessness, word articulation, tongue protrusion, and facial aesthetics.

Although the small sample sized used in this study is not sufficient to create general guidelines, it is hopeful that the promising results of this study will prompt further investigation into this area.

AIRWAY ABNORMALITIES IN PATIENTS WITH DOWN SYNDROME

In addition to OSA, patients with Down syndrome have anomalies of the upper and lower airway that, combined with comorbidities such as GERD, hypotonia, and obesity, may create complex and chronic large airway obstruction. A review of all patients referred to a tertiary care center in New Mexico during a 2.5-year period for upper airway obstruction showed that the most common reason for referral was laryngomalacia (43%), with most of these patients being less than 1 month old.[87] Laryngomalacia is more common in children with neurologic disorders, particularly hypotonia.

Generalized Hypotonia

Patients with Down syndrome have generalized hypotonia, leading to flaccidity of the supraglottis; anatomic changes in the epiglottis, arytenoids, and aryepiglottic folds; and a high prevalence of GERD. Severe laryngomalacia can usually be surgically corrected by aryepiglottoplasty, which is safe and effective in children without significant comorbidities.[88] We know of no published data on the outcomes of aryepiglottoplasty in patients with Down syndrome; however, the generalized hypotonia, the high incidence of GERD, and the likelihood of multiple intubations for further surgical procedures make this a more complicated procedure in the patient with Down syndrome. It is therefore recommended that patients be referred to tertiary care centers that are familiar with the requirements of these patients.

A review of all patients with Down syndrome with upper airway obstruction over 5 years at Egleston Children's Hospital shows the complexity of these patients and the multifactorial nature of their disease, and shows the treatment challenges.[89] In the study by Jacobs and colleagues,[89] 71 of 518 patients with Down syndrome were diagnosed with airway obstruction. Of these 71, the 39 who had the most severe symptoms underwent operative endoscopy including flexible fiberoptic endoscopy, rigid laryngoscopy, and bronchoscopy. Outcomes for the 39 patients following laryngoscopy and bronchoscopy were:

- Multiple sites of obstruction were seen in 38% of cases
- Tracheomalacia was found in 23 of 39 (59%)
- Laryngomalacia in 28%
- Macroglossia in 26%
- Subglottic stenosis in 23%
- Congenital tracheal stenosis in 5%.

In this study, children with severe symptoms were more likely to be younger and have more than 1 site of airway obstruction. Nearly one-quarter of the patients in this study had residual symptoms after surgical correction, likely caused by the severe baseline degree of obstruction, multiple anatomic sites of obstruction, and craniofacial structural problems. Again, it is important that these cases be managed by a tertiary care center experienced with treating patients with Down syndrome and practiced at comprehensive airway evaluations and a systemic approach to surgery in children with Down syndrome. Even at centers with a high volume of patients with Down syndrome, parents should be counseled before surgery about the possibility of residual symptoms in children with severe obstruction.

Subglottic Stenosis

Subglottic stenosis is also thought to be more prevalent in the Down syndrome population, although the exact prevalence and cause is difficult to determine. A study reviewing laryngotracheal reconstruction (LTR) showed that 4% of LTRs done at that hospital were on patients with Down syndrome.[90] The prevalence of Down syndrome is 0.1% to 0.15% of live births, so they concluded that subglottic stenosis may be more common in patients with Down syndrome. The higher prevalence is likely caused by a higher incidence of congenital narrowing of the subglottis as well acquired deformities. A retrospective review of 15 patients with Down syndrome who underwent laryngotracheoplasty for subglottic stenosis found the risk factor for subglottic stenosis in children with Down syndrome to be the same in the Down syndrome group as for the general population; trauma to the subglottis.[91] The child with Down syndrome has a higher rate of major surgery (ie, cardiac anomalies) and intubation, as well as severe respiratory infections requiring intubation.[82] In patients with Down syndrome, this usually occurs at a young age, which predisposes them to subglottic injury and, subsequently, subglottic stenosis. Therefore, subglottic stenosis is more commonly seen in the Down syndrome population.[23] One study of 99 patients with Down syndrome who underwent cardiovascular surgery found that 24 (24.2%) of the patients had postextubation stridor, and subglottic stenosis was found in 6 (6.1%).[92] In the 6 who had subglottic stenosis, all 6 were at less than the 10th percentile for weight, and an endotracheal tube of a larger diameter than expected for age was used in 4 patients.

Endotracheal Tube Selection for the Child with Down Syndrome

A key factor in preventing subglottic injury is choosing an appropriate-sized endotracheal tube, because age-appropriate endotracheal tubes are too large for the patient with Down syndrome. One retrospective study reviewed 100 patients with Down syndrome undergoing endotracheal intubation.[93] Of these 100 patients with Down syndrome, 20 required endotracheal tubes smaller than their expected age, leading to the conclusion that the airway in the patient with Down syndrome is inherently smaller. A prospective study evaluated 74 children, 42 with Down syndrome and 32 healthy controls, none of whom had wheezing, stridor, or previous intubation before surgery.[94] The children with Down syndrome required an endotracheal tube 2 to 3 sizes smaller than age-matched controls. Further, MRI showed that tracheal diameter was smaller in Down syndrome compared with controls, showing that the overall smaller airway size is not limited to the subglottis, but includes a smaller trachea. In any surgery, the appropriate-sized endotracheal tube should be used. In children with Down syndrome, it is important to be aware that age-appropriate endotracheal tubes may be too large, and it is important to check for an appropriate air leak around the endotracheal tube. Based on this prospective study, it is recommended that endotracheal tubes at least 2 sizes smaller should initially be used for intubation in children with Down syndrome.[92] To ensure proper-sized tube placement, it is critical to confirm the fit of the tube after it is placed by checking for an audible air leak at an inspiratory pressure between 10 and 30 cm H_2O.

ANESTHESIA CONSIDERATIONS AND COMORBIDITIES IN PATIENTS WITH DOWN SYNDROME

In addition to the special needs for intubation and endotracheal tube selection, children with Down syndrome are at higher risk for other complications of anesthesia.

Complications from Atlantoaxial Instability

One consideration that the otolaryngologist must take into account is atlantoaxial instability (AAI). Although AAI is one of the most well-known and feared problems associated with Down syndrome, reports of complications associated with AAI are few, and current guidelines and recommendations of airway management and positioning during surgery for the patients are vague. Studies have shown that the incidence of AAI seen on radiography is 14% to 20%.[9,95] However, the incidence of symptomatic AAI is much less, with only a few case reports throughout the literature. In the study of 404 patients with Down syndrome that found 14.6% to have radiographic evidence of AAI, only 1.5% of the patients had symptoms.[94] Atlantoaxial instability, also called atlantoaxial subluxation, is the result of increased mobility at the articulation of the first and second cervical vertebrae.

A review reports that craniocervical instability, most commonly atlantoaxial instability, is the result of generalized ligamentous laxity, involving any of the 3 ligaments of the C1C2 joint. It can be acquired or precipitated by upper respiratory infections. Rotation of the head may result in C1C2 subluxation.[96]

Atlantoaxial Instability: Imaging Studies

The radiographic definition of AAI is made by measuring the distance between the anterior surface of the dens to the posterior surface of the tubercle of C1. An anterior atlantodental interval of greater than 4.5 indicates abnormal instability. Asymptomatic AAI is AAI that is diagnosed by radiography, but the patient has no neurologic symptoms.

The patient who is symptomatic may experience (**Fig. 6**):

- Easy fatiguability
- Abnormal gait and difficulty walking
- Neck pain
- Limited neck mobility
- Torticollis
- Clumsiness
- Lack of coordination
- Sensory deficits
- Spasticity
- Hyperreflexia
- Clonus
- Incontinence
- Extensor-plantar reflex.

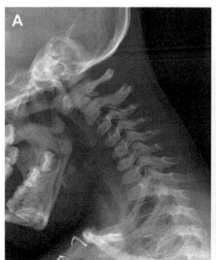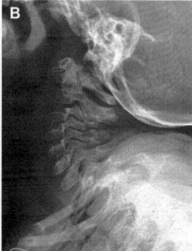

Fig. 6. (*A*) Patient with Down syndrome in flexion. Note the change in the atlantodens interval between flexion and extension in (*B; red arrows*). Also note the change in the posterior atlantodens interval, also known as the space available for cord (*blue arrow*), between the 2 films.

The issue of atlantoaxial instability came to wide recognition after the Special Olympics introduced a requirement in 1983 that all individuals with Down syndrome have a lateral neck radiograph before participating, and that those with evidence of instability be banned from certain activities. This requirement was further supported by a statement by the American Academy of Pediatrics (AAP) in 1984.[97] Since these statements were issued, more research has been done on the subject, bringing evidence that radiographic screening is not the best method to prevent injury from AAI.

One report prospectively studied 135 children with Down syndrome to find clinical predictors of symptomatic AAI, and found that abnormal gait was the only significant clinical predictor of adverse outcome, and that radiographs of the neck were unreliable at identifying atlantoaxial subluxation.[98] A review by the AAP of case reports of individuals who have experienced catastrophic injury to the spinal cord determined that trauma rarely causes the initial symptoms or progression of symptoms, and that nearly all the individuals who have experienced catastrophic injury to the spinal cord had weeks to years of preceding, less severe, neurologic abnormalities.[9,94,99,100]

Atlantoaxial Instability: Physical Examination and History

In a 1995 statement, the AAP retired their previous statement, and revised their recommendations to state that evaluation and physical examination by a physician who has cared for the patient longitudinally is a greater priority than obtaining radiographs when determining the eligibility of a patient with Down syndrome for participation in sports.[101] It is now recommended that the pediatrician perform a careful history and physical examination with attention to myelopathic signs and symptoms at every well-child visit, or when symptoms possibly attributable to spinal cord impingement are reported.[35]

Somatosensory Evoked Potentials in Patients with Down Syndrome

The 1980s focus on atlantoaxial instability by the Special Olympics and AAP raised concerns by otolaryngologists, who frequently perform surgery in nonneutral neck positions. At least 1 case of quadriplegia attributed to atlantoaxial subluxation during ear surgery has been reported.[102] Recently, investigation into using somatosensory evoked potentials (SEPs) to prevent spinal cord injury has been performed. The SEP measures the speed and efficiency of afferent neural transmission and processing. A delay in SEP latency suggests spinal cord compression. In one study, 17 patients with Down syndrome, who were undergoing elective otolaryngologic surgery, with no evidence of C-spine problem by neurologic examination and had an atlantodens interval of less than 5 mm by radiography, had SEP monitoring during surgery. In each patient, the head was rotated 60° right and 60° left. In all cases, the patients maintained normal SEPs. The conclusion of this study is that patients with Down syndrome who are neurologically intact and who have normal lateral neck radiographs, with more than 99.99% certainty, do not seem to be at great risk with neck rotation, as would be performed in ear surgery. As the use of SEP continues to be studied and developed, it may become routine for use in cases involving patients with Down syndrome. There is currently not enough evidence to include SEP in guidelines. Because of the poor ability of radiographs to detect clinical neurologic compromise, it is imperative that every patient have a thorough neurologic examination before surgery, preferably by a physician who knows the patient well. Although gentle rotation of the head for ear surgery is likely safe, it is still recommended that the patient's head be supported throughout the procedure, and that extremes of neck positioning be avoided. When performing tonsillectomy, the patient should remain in a neutral position (**Fig. 7**).

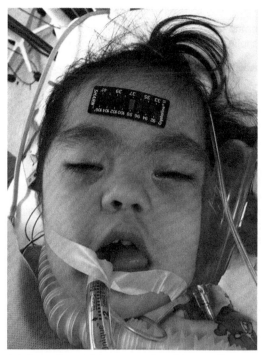

Fig. 7. It is important to keep the neck in a neutral position at all times. An anesthesia mask can be used to support the head during ear surgery.

GERD in Patients with Down Syndrome

Another comorbidity found with high prevalence in the Down syndrome population that is of particular interest to the otolaryngologist is GERD. A study reviewing all patients with Down syndrome referred to a tertiary care center found systemic comorbidities in 93% of patients, with GERD being the most common, diagnosed in 59%.[103] Ear, nose, and throat disease is exacerbated by GERD.[104] In a study of laryngotracheoplasty in Down syndrome, in addition to a high incidence of subglottic stenosis, there was also a higher rate of postglottic stenosis within patients with Down syndrome compared with the overall series.[90] Of the patients who were tested for GERD, 9 of 9 were found to be positive. The authors of this study think that GERD is a contributing factor in forming subglottic stenosis, and, in the face of previous mucosal injury, acid reflux may encourage scar formation in the posterior glottis. In addition, failure to control reflux can interfere with graft healing.[90] It is imperative that the otolaryngologist diagnoses and aggressively manages GERD in the patient with Down syndrome.

Cardiac and Other Anesthetic Considerations in Patients with Down Syndrome

There are other anesthetic considerations of patients with Down syndrome:

- Cardiac lesions
- Conductive disturbances
- Pulmonary hypertension
- Polycythemia in neonates

- Hypothyroidism
- Sensitivity to atropine
- Decreased catecholamine release, resulting in deeper levels of anesthesia.

A full discussion of these comorbidities is beyond the scope of this article. It is important for the surgeon to obtain all past medical and surgical history and to ensure that all members of the surgical team are familiar with the patient's history and that proper precautions are taken. Communication between the anesthesiologist, surgeon, and operating room team is key to successful outcomes.

SUMMARY ON OTOLARYNGOLOGIC CARE OF CHILDREN WITH DOWN SYNDROME

As children with Down syndrome live longer, and become integrated into mainstream society, more emphasis is being placed on quality of life and using health care to help these children maximize their potential. It is likely that most children with Down syndrome will be seen by an otolaryngologist at some point.

- For stenotic ear canals and cerumen impaction, pediatricians should not hesitate to refer the child to an otolaryngologist for cerumen removal and microscopic examination.
- The child with Down syndrome should undergo behavioral audiologic testing every 6 months, or every 3 months if the patient has very stenotic ear canals. This behavioral audiologic testing should continue until the child is able to cooperate with ear-specific testing.
- Treatment of recurrent otitis media and OME should be aggressive and postoperative results should be closely followed with serial physical examinations and audiometry.
- Parents should be prepared for multiple sets of PE tubes throughout the child's life.
- Patients with Down syndrome have a higher prevalence of OSA than nonsyndromic children. The consequence of untreated OSA is hypoxemia and hypoventilation, and this can lead to development of pulmonary hypertension and congestive heart failure. Because it has been shown that parents are not reliable predictors of sleep apnea, it is recommended that all children with Down syndrome get polysomnography between the ages of 3 and 4 years.
- Primary treatment of OSAS is tonsillectomy and adenoidectomy, but parents should be prepared that this is curative in only 25% of children, and that their child may require further surgery to alleviate obstruction.
- Treatment of chronic rhinitis and sinusitis should be aggressive and include saline nasal spray, antihistamines, decongestants, nasal steroids, and antibiotics if needed.
- Airway anomalies are more common in the Down syndrome population, with subglottic stenosis being more prevalent than in the general population. Prevention of subglottic stenosis can be achieved in part by using an endotracheal tube 2 sizes smaller than predicted for the patient's age, and ensuring that an audible air leak is present around the tube.
- In cases of complex airway trauma requiring surgical repair, these are better managed at a tertiary care center with experience in syndromic children, because of the high rate of complications in these patients.
- Because of the high prevalence of GERD in this population and the effect it can have on otolaryngologic disease, all patients with Down syndrome should be evaluated for GERD and aggressively treated if it is found to be present.

To the pediatrician caring for children with Down syndrome

Stenotic ear canals: patients with Down syndrome often have stenotic ear canals. These narrowed canals predispose the patient with Down syndrome to cerumen impaction, and the cerumen combined with the stenotic canal make it difficult to adequately examine the ear. Further, it has been observed that patients with stenotic ear canals had an increased incidence of associated middle ear effusions. If it is difficult to examine the ear in the office, patients should be referred to an otolaryngologist early for microscopic examination and cerumen disimpaction of the canals under microscopy.

Otitis media and hearing loss: children with Down syndrome are predisposed to serous otitis media and resulting conductive hearing loss. Hearing impairment may be masked in patients with intellectual impairment, because speech delays and lack of response to verbal cues may be attributed to mental retardation. However, detection of this loss is critical, because the detrimental effects of hearing loss on language development are thought to be greater for those children with learning disabilities compared with children without mental retardation. Therefore, it is recommended that all children with Down syndrome go for routine audiologic screening. The AAP Committee on Genetic and the Down Syndrome Interest Group Guideline recommend audiologic testing at birth, then every 6 months up to age 3 years, with annual testing after 3 years of age, or when pure tone audiometry may be obtained.

Pressure equalization tube placement: patients with Down syndrome with recurrent otitis media and effusion should be referred to the otolaryngologist early in life for PE tube placement. Parents should be counseled that PE tubes may be placed earlier in the child's life, and to expect that the child may need multiple set of tubes throughout childhood, even into adulthood.

Obstructive sleep apnea: children with Down syndrome have many predisposing factors of OSAS. These factors include midfacial and mandibular hypoplasia, glossoptosis, an abnormally small upper airway with superficially positioned tonsils and relative tonsillar and adenoidal encroachment, increased secretions, and increased incidence of lower respiratory tract anomalies, obesity, and generalized hypotonia with resultant collapse of the airway during inspiration. OSAS can lead to heart failure secondary to the chronic, intermittent hypoxemia and respiratory acidosis during sleep.

Polysomnography: it may be difficult for a parent to tell whether a child is suffering from sleep apnea, because the most severe apneic events often happen during REM sleep, late at night, when the parents are also asleep. In the child with Down syndrome, the parent may assume that the child's irregular breathing at night is normal for a child with Down syndrome, which is a frequently expressed comment. It is recommended that all children with Down syndrome between the ages of 3 and 4 years go for objective testing using full overnight polysomnography for a baseline study.

Tonsillectomy and adenoidectomy: patients with Down syndrome with OSAS should be referred to the otolaryngologist for tonsillectomy and adenoidectomy, which is the initial treatment of OSAS; however, parents should be counseled that the efficacy of tonsillectomy and adenoidectomy in curing sleep apnea in patients with Down syndrome is generally accepted to be lower than in the general pediatric population, with 30% to 50% of patients with Down syndrome requiring CPAP support, further surgery, or tracheostomy at a later date.

Chronic rhinitis and sinusitis: the patient with Down syndrome is predisposed to chronic nasal drainage, nasal obstruction, and sinusitis caused by the narrowing of the nose and nasal sinuses. The narrowing of the nasopharynx leads normal growth of adenoid tissue to obstruct the airway, predisposing patients to nasal congestion and subsequent infection. Several studies have shown abnormalities in the Ig levels. Treatment of this nasal drainage is similar to the general population, with nasal irrigation, nasal steroids, antihistamines, decongestants, and antibiotics as needed.

Several studies have shown that GERD is common in the Down syndrome pediatric population, diagnosed in 59% of patients with Down syndrome in 1 study. It is known that ear, nose, and throat disease is exacerbated by GERD. It is important that the pediatrician evaluate the patient for GERD and ensures aggressive treatment.

- During surgery in patients with Down syndrome, the surgeon should always be aware of the possibility of atlantoaxial instability, and no dramatic head movement should be made. In tonsillectomy, the patient's head should remain in a neutral position, and, during otologic surgery, the patient's head may be turned, but should be supported at all times.
- After surgery, patients with Down syndrome tend to have a higher rate of complications including stridor, desaturations, poor oral intake, and behavioral problems. Because of this, it is recommended that children with Down syndrome be admitted for observation when intubation is required, even for short procedures such as tonsillectomy and adenoidectomy.

Although these children have disease that is more complex and difficult to treat than the nonsyndromic pediatric patient, the general otolaryngologist can have a profound impact on the patient with Down syndrome. Proper management of ear, nose, and throat disorders by the otolaryngologist can support the physical, emotional, and educational development of the child with Down syndrome.

REFERENCES

1. Centers for Disease Control and Prevention (CDC). Down syndrome prevalence at birth: United States, 1983-1990. MMWR Morb Mortal Wkly Rep 1994;43: 617–22.
2. Yang Q, Rasmussen S, Friedman J. Mortality associated with Down's syndrome in the USA from 1983 to 1997: a population based study. Lancet 2002;359:1019–25.
3. Roizen NJ, Patterson D. Down's syndrome. Lancet 2003;361:1281–9.
4. Bittles AH, Bower C, Hussain R, et al. The four ages of Down syndrome. Eur J Public Health 2007;17(2):221–5.
5. Hans PS, Belloso A, Sheehan PZ. Parental satisfaction with health services provided to children with Down syndrome in north-west England: an ENT perspective. J Laryngol Otol 2006;121:382–6.
6. Shibahara Y, Sando I. Congenital anomalies of the Eustachian tube in children with Down syndrome. Ann Otol Rhinol Laryngol 1989;98:543–7.
7. Austin J, Preger L, Siris E, et al. Short hard palate in newborn: roentgen sign of mongolism. Radiology 1969;92:775–6.
8. Strome M. Obstructive sleep apnea in Down's syndrome: a surgical approach. Laryngoscope 1986;96:1340–2.
9. Miller J, Capusten B, Lampard R. Changes at the base of the skull and cervical spine in Down syndrome. J Can Assoc Radiol 1986;37:85–9.
10. Gershwin ME, Crinella FM, Castles JJ, et al. Immunologic characteristics of Down's syndrome. J Ment Defic Res 1977;21:237–48.
11. Kovesi T, Sinclair B, MacCormick J, et al. Primary ciliary dyskinesia associated with Down syndrome. Chest 2000;117:1207–9.
12. Sonek J, Cicero S, Neiger R, et al. Nasal bone assessment in prenatal screening for trisomy 21. Am J Obstet Gynecol 2006;195:1219–30.
13. Prefumo F, Sairam S, Bhide A, et al. First trimester nuchal translucency, nasal bones, and trisomy 21 in selected and unselected populations. Am J Obstet Gynecol 2006;194:828–33.
14. Sonek J, Nicolaides K. Additional first-trimester ultrasound markers. Clin Lab Med 2010;30:573–92.
15. Nicolaides KH. Screening for fetal aneuploidies at 11-13 weeks. Prenat Diagn 2011;31(1):7–15.

16. Cicero S, Sonek JD, McKenna DS, et al. Nasal bone hypoplasia in trisomy 21 at 15-22 weeks gestation. Ultrasound Obstet Gynecol 2003;21(1):15–8.
17. Miguelez J, Moskovitch M, Cuckle H, et al. Model-predicted performance of second-trimester Down syndrome screening with sonographic prenasal thickness. J Ultrasound Med 2010;29:1741–7.
18. Ting YH, Lao T, Lau TK, et al. Isolated absent or hypoplastic nasal bone in the second trimester fetus: is amniocentesis necessary? J Matern Fetal Neonatal Med 2011;24(4):555–8.
19. Strome M. Down's syndrome-a modern otorhinolaryngological perspective. Laryngoscope 1981;42:1581–94.
20. Shott SR. Down syndrome: common otolaryngologic manifestations. Am J Med Genet C Semin Med Genet 2006;142C:131–40.
21. Cunningham C, McArthur K. Hearing loss and treatment in young Downs syndrome children. Child Care Health Dev 1982;7:357–74.
22. Selikowitz M. Health problems and health checks in school aged children with Down syndrome. J Paediatr Child Health 1992;28:383–6.
23. Chaushu S, Yefenof E, Becker A, et al. A link between parotid salivary Ig level and recurrent respiratory infections in young Down's syndrome patients. Oral Microbiol Immunol 2002;17:172–6.
24. Nespoli L, Burgio GR, Ugazio AG, et al. Immunological feature of Down's syndrome: a review. J Intellect Disabil Res 1993;37:543–51.
25. Brown PM, Lewis GT, Parker AJ, et al. The skull base and nasopharynx in relation in Down's syndrome in relation to hearing impairment. Clin Otolaryngol 1989;14:241–6.
26. Yamaguchi N, Sando I, Hashida Y, et al. Histologic study of eustachian tube cartilage with and without congenital anomalies: a preliminary study. Ann Otol Rhinol Laryngol 1990;99:984–7.
27. Han F, Yu H, Zhang J, et al. Otitis media in a mouse model for Down syndrome. Int J Exp Pathol 2009;90:480–8.
28. McPherson B, Lai S, Leung K, et al. Hearing loss in Chinese school children with Down syndrome. Int J Pediatr Otorhinolaryngol 2007;71:1905–15.
29. Krecicki T, Zalesska-Krecicka M, Kubiak K, et al. Brain auditory potentials in children with Down syndrome. Int J Pediatr Otorhinolaryngol 2005;69(5):615–20.
30. Hess C, Rosanowski F, Eysholdt U, et al. Hearing impairment in children and adolescents with Down syndrome. HNO 2006;54(3):227–32.
31. Harigai S. Longitudinal studies in hearing-impaired children with Down syndrome. Nippon Jibiinkoka Gakkai Kaiho 1994;97(12):2208–18.
32. Balkany TJ, Dows MP, Jafek BW, et al. Hearing loss in Downs syndrome: a treatable handicap more common than generally recognized. Clin Pediatr 1979;18:116–8.
33. Downs MP. The hearing of Downs individuals. Seminars in Speech, Language and Hearing 1980;1:25–37.
34. Cohen WI. Health care guidelines for individuals with Down Syndrome. Down Syndrome Quarterly 1999;4(3):1–16.
35. Bull M, AAP Committee on Genetics. AAP clinical report: health supervision for children with Down syndrome. Pediatrics 2011;128(2):393–406.
36. Maw R, Bawden R. Spontaneous resolution of severe chronic glue ear in children and the effect of adenoidectomy, tonsillectomy and insertion of ventilation tubes (grommets). BMJ 1993;306:756–60.
37. Selikowitz M. Short term efficacy of tympanostomy tubes for secretory otitis media in children with Down syndrome. Dev Med Child Neurol 1993;35:511–5.

38. Iino Y, Imamura Y, Harigai S, et al. Efficacy of tympanostomy tube insertion for otitis media with effusion in children with Down syndrome. Int J Pediatr Otorhinolaryngol 1999;49:143–9.

39. Bluestone CD, Kein JO. Otitis media in infants and children. 2nd edition. Philadelphia: Saunders; 1995.

40. Iino Y, Imamura Y, Haigai S, et al. Clinical course of otitis media with effusion in child with Down syndrome: recent advances in otitis media. Hamilton (ON): Decker; 1996. p. 52–3.

41. Davies B, Land D, Stratford B. Hearing problems in Down syndrome: current approaches to Down syndrome. London: Cassell. p. 85–102.

42. Shott SR, Joseph A, Heithaus D. Hearing loss in children with Down syndrome. Int J Pediatr Otorhinolaryngol 2001;61:199–205.

43. Whiteman B, Simpson G, Compton W. Relationship of otitis media and language impairment in adolescents with Down syndrome. Ment Retard 1986;24(6): 353–6.

44. Blaser S, Propst E, Martin D, et al. Inner ear dysplasia is common in children with Down syndrome (trisomy 21). Laryngoscope 2006;116:2113–9.

45. Glass RB, Yousefzadeh DK, Roizen NJ. Mastoid abnormalities in Down syndrome. Pediatr Radiol 1989;19:311–2.

46. Balkany T, Mischke R, Downs M, et al. Ossicular abnormalities in Downs syndrome. Otolaryngol Head Neck Surg 1979;87:372–84.

47. O'Malley M, Kaylie D, Himbergen D, et al. Chronic ear surgery in patients with syndromes and multiple congenital malformations. Laryngoscope 2007;117: 1993–8.

48. Bacciu A, Pasanisi E, Vincenti V, et al. Surgical treatment of middle ear cholesteatoma in children with Down syndrome. Otol Neurotol 2005;26:1007–10.

49. Sheehan P, Hans P. UK and Ireland experience of bone anchored hearing aids (BAHA) in individuals with Down syndrome. Int J Pediatr Otorhinolaryngol 2006; 70:981–6.

50. McDermott A, Williams J, Kuo M, et al. The role of bone anchored hearing aids in children with Down syndrome. Int J Pediatr Otorhinolaryngol 2008;72:751–7.

51. Watson GJ, Sheehan PZ. A Protective cage for the post operative care of the skin graft and wound of the BAHA site in patients with Down syndrome and other learning disabilities. Clin Otolaryngol 2008;33(1):73–4.

52. Hans PS, England R, Prowse S, et al. UK and Ireland experience of cochlear implants in children with Down syndrome. Int J Pediatr Otorhinolaryngol 2010; 74:260–4.

53. Pappas D, Flexer C, Shackelford L. Otological and habilitative management of children with Down syndrome. Laryngoscope 1994;104(9):1065–70.

54. Bennetts L, Flynn M. Improving the classroom listening skills of children with Down syndrome by using sound field amplification. Downs Syndr Res Pract 2002;8(1):19–24.

55. Ali NJ, Pitson DJ, Strandling JR. Snoring, sleep disturbance, and behavior in 4-5 year olds. Arch Dis Child 1993;68:360–6.

56. Gislason T, Benediktsdottir B. Snoring, apneic episodes, and nocturnal hypoxemia among children 6 months to 6 years old. Chest 1995;107:963–6.

57. Marcus C, Keens T, Bautista D, et al. Obstructive sleep apnea in children with Down syndrome. Pediatrics 1991;88(1):132–9.

58. Shott S, Amin R, Chini B, et al. Obstructive sleep apnea: should all children with Down syndrome be tested? Arch Otolaryngol Head Neck Surg 2006;132: 432–6.

59. Fink GB, Madaus WK, Walker GF. A quantitative study of the face in Downs syndrome. Am J Orthod 1975;67:540–53.
60. Beebe DW, Wells CT, Jeffries J, et al. Neuropsychological effects of pediatric obstructive sleep apnea. J Int Neuropsychol Soc 2004;10:962–75.
61. Brouillette RT, Fernbach SK, Hunt CE. Obstructive sleep apnea in infants and children. J Pediatr 1982;100:31–40.
62. Perkin RM, Anas NG. Pulmonary hypertension in pediatric patients. J Pediatr 1984;105:511–22.
63. Hals J, Hagemo PS, Thaulow E, et al. Pulmonary vascular resistance in complete atrioventricular septal defect: a comparison between children with and without Downs syndrome. Acta Pediatrica 1993;82:595–8.
64. Fitzgerald D, Paul A, Richmond C. Severity of obstructive sleep apnoea in children with Down syndrome who snore. Arch Dis Child 2007;92:423–5.
65. Sutherland K, Lee RW, Phillips CL, et al. Effect of weight loss on upper airway size in facial fat in men with obstructive sleep apnoea. Thorax 2011;66(9):797–803.
66. Dyken M, Lin Dykin D, Poulton M, et al. Prospective polysomnographic analysis of obstruction sleep apnea in Down syndrome. Arch Pediatr Adolesc Med 2003; 157:655–60.
67. Shires C, Anold S, Schoumacher R, et al. Body mass index as an indicator of obstructive sleep apnea in pediatric Down syndrome. Int J Pediatr Otorhinolaryngol 2010;74:768–72.
68. Must A, Anderson SE. Body mass index in children and adolescents: considerations for population-based applications. Int J Obes 2006;30:590–4.
69. Roland P, Rosenfield R, Brooks L, et al. Polysomnography for sleep disordered breathing prior to tonsillectomy in children. Otolaryngol Head Neck Surg 2011; 145(1):S1–15.
70. Mitchell RB. Adenotonsillectomy for obstructive sleep apnea in children: outcome evaluated by pre-and postoperative polysomnography. Laryngoscope 2007;117(10):1844–54.
71. Donnelly L, Shott S, LaRose C, et al. Causes of persistent obstructive sleep apnea despite previous tonsillectomy and adenoidectomy in children with Down syndrome as depicted on static and dynamic cine MRI. AJR Am J Roentgenol 1994;183:175–81.
72. Shete M, Stocks R, Sebelik M, et al. Effects of adeno-tonsillectomy on polysomnography patterns in Down syndrome children with obstructive sleep apnea: a comparative study with children without Down syndrome. Int J Pediatr Otorhinolaryngol 2010;74:241–4.
73. Merrell J, Shott S. OSAS in Down syndrome: T&A versus T&A plus lateral pharyngoplasty. Int J Pediatr Otorhinolaryngol 2007;71:1197–203.
74. Freidman M, Wilson M, Lin LC, et al. Updated systemic review of tonsillectomy and adenoidectomy for treatment of pediatric obstructive sleep apnea/hypopnea syndrome. Otolaryngol Head Neck Surg 2009;140:800–8.
75. Wolkove N, Blatzan M, Kamel H, et al. Long term compliance with continuous positive pressure airway pressure in Patients with obstructive sleep apnea. Can Respir J 2008;15(7):365–9.
76. Kavanagn K, Kahane J, Kordan B. Risks and benefits of adenotonsillectomy for children with Down syndrome. Am J Ment Defic 1986;91(1):22–9.
77. Gelder LV. Open nasal speech following adenoidectomy and tonsillectomy. J Commun Dis 1974;4:263–7.
78. Gibb AG. Hypernasality (rhinolalia aperta) following tonsil and adenoid removal. J Laryngol Otol 1958;72:433–51.

79. Goldstein N, Armfield D, Kingsley L, et al. Postoperative complications after tonsillectomy and adenoidectomy in children with Down syndrome. Arch Otolaryngol Head Neck Surg 1998;124:171–6.

80. Caulfield H. Investigations in pediatric obstructive sleep apnea: do we need them? Int J Pediatr Otorhinolaryngol 2003;67S1:S107–10.

81. Shott S, Donnelly L. Cine magnetic resonance imaging: evaluation of persistent airway obstruction after tonsil and adenoidectomy in children with Down syndrome. Laryngoscope 2004;114:1724–9.

82. Wootten C, Shott S. Evolving therapies to treat retroglossal and base of tongue obstruction in pediatric obstructive sleep apnea. Arch Otolaryngol Head Neck Surg 2010;136(10):983–7.

83. Chaushu S, Chaushu G, Zigmond M, et al. Age-dependency in saliva and salivary secretion in Downs syndrome. Arch Oral Biol 2007;52(11):1088–96.

84. Chaushu S, Yefe Nof E, Becker A, et al. Parotid salivary immunoglobulins, recurrent respiratory tract infections and gingival health in institutionalized and non-institutionalized subjects with Down's syndrome. J Intellect Disabil Res 2003; 47:101–7.

85. Moura CP, Andrade D, Cunha LM, et al. Down syndrome: otolaryngological effects of rapid maxillary expansion. J Laryngol Otol 2008;122:1318–24.

86. Moura CP, Andrade D, Cunha LM, et al. Rapid maxillary expansion and nasal patency in children with Down syndrome. Rhinology 2005;43:138–42.

87. Mitchell R, Call E, Kelly J. Diagnosis and therapy for airway obstruction in children with Down syndrome. Arch Otolaryngol Head Neck Surg 2003;129: 642–5.

88. Roger G, Denoyelle F, Triglia J, et al. Severe laryngomalacia: surgical indications and results in 115 patients. Laryngoscope 1995;105:1111–7.

89. Jacobs I, Gray R, Todd W. Upper airway obstruction in children with Down syndrome. Arch Otolaryngol Head Neck Surg 1996;22:945–50.

90. Miller R, Gray S, Cotton R, et al. Subglottic stenosis and Down syndrome. Am J Otolaryngol 1990;11:274–7.

91. Boseley M, Link D, Shott S, et al. Laryngotracheoplasty for subglottic stenosis in Down syndrome children: the Cincinnati experience. Int J Pediatr Otorhinolaryngol 2001;57:11–5.

92. De Long AL, Sulek M, Nihill M, et al. Tenuous airway in children with trisomy 21. Laryngoscope 1997;107:345–9.

93. Kobel M, Creighton RE, Steward DJ. Anaesthetic considerations in Downs syndrome: with 100 patients and a review of the literature. Can Anaesth Soc J 1982;29:393–8.

94. Shott SR. Down syndrome: analysis of airway size and guide for appropriate intubation. Laryngoscope 2000;110:585–92.

95. Pueschel S, Scola F. Atlantoaxial instability in individuals with Down syndrome: epidemiologic, radiographic, and clinical studies. Pediatrics 1987;80(4): 555–60.

96. Bhattarai B, Kulkarni H, Kalingarayar S, et al. Anesthetic management of a child with Down's syndrome having atlanto-axial instability. JNMA J Nepal Med Assoc 2009;48(173):66–9.

97. American Academy of Pediatrics, Committee on Sports Medicine. Atlantoaxial instability in Down syndrome. Pediatrics 1984;74:152–4.

98. Selby K, Newton R, Gupta S, et al. Clinical predictors and radiological reliability in atlantoaxial subluxation in Downs syndrome. Arch Dis Child 1991; 66:876–8.

99. Riaz S, Drake J, Hedden D. Images in spine surgery: atlantoaxial instability in Down syndrome. J Pak Med Assoc 2007;57(4):213–4.
100. Hreidarsson S, Magram G, Singer H. Symptomatic atlantoaxial dislocation in Down syndrome. Pediatrics 1982;69(5):568–71.
101. American Academy of Pediatrics, Committee on Sports Medicine and Fitness. Atlantoaxial instability in Down syndrome: subject review. Pediatrics 1995;96: 151–4.
102. Litman RS, Perkins FM. Atlantoaxial subluxation after tympanomastoidectomy in a child with trisomy 21. Otolaryngol Head Neck Surg 1994;110:584–6.
103. Mitchell R, Call E, Kelly J. Ear, nose and throat disorders in children with Down syndrome. Laryngoscope 2003;113:259–63.
104. Suskind D, Zeringue G, Kluka E, et al. Gastroesophageal reflux and pediatric otolaryngologic disease: the role of anti reflux surgery. Arch Otolaryngol Head Neck Surg 2001;127:511–4.

Allergic Fungal Sinusitis in Children

Brian D. Thorp, MD[a], Kibwei A. McKinney, MD[a],
Austin S. Rose, MD[a], Charles S. Ebert Jr, MD, MPH[a,b,*]

KEYWORDS

- Pediatric sinusitis • Pediatric rhinosinusitis • Allergic fungal sinusitis
- Management of rhinosinusitis • Chronic rhinosinusitis

KEY POINTS

- Allergic fungal sinusitis (AFS) is a distinct subtype of eosinophilic CRS marked by type I hypersensitivity (by history, skin tests, or serology), nasal polyposis, characteristic computed tomography findings, eosinophilic mucus, and the presence of fungal elements of the tissue removed during surgery without evidence of fungal tissue invasion.
- AFS is most common among adolescents and young adults.
- The treatment of AFS is both medical and surgical.
- Functional endoscopic sinus surgery is the intervention of choice in this patient population, as nearly all cases of AFS will require some form of surgical management.
- Active postoperative care is crucial to the successful management of these patients, and can reduce the need for further surgical procedures.

▶ TWO VIDEOS ACCOMPANY THIS ARTICLE: ONE VIDEO DEMONSTRATES AFS NASAL POLY REMOVAL AND THE OTHER DEMONSTRATES FESS for AFS AT http://www.oto.theclinics.com/.

Chronic rhinosinusitis (CRS) is a complex, heterogeneous disease process that affects nearly 37 million people in the United States each year and accounts for approximately $6 billion in direct and indirect health care costs.[1] Estimates indicate that sinusitis is more widespread than arthritis or hypertension, and its effects on quality of life are comparable to that of many chronic debilitating diseases.[2] Despite its substantial impact on quality of life and financial burden to the health care system, little is known about the etiology and pathophysiology. Moreover, controversy regarding appropriate treatment options remains. This lack of consensus pertains to the adult population but

Disclosures: None.
[a] Department of Otolaryngology-Head and Neck Surgery, University of North Carolina School of Medicine, Campus Box #7070, Chapel Hill, NC 27599-7070, USA; [b] Division of Rhinology, Allergy, and Endoscopic Skull Base Surgery, Department of Otolaryngology-Head and Neck Surgery, University of North Carolina School of Medicine, Chapel Hill, NC, USA
* Corresponding author. Department of Otolaryngology-Head & Neck Surgery, University of North Carolina School of Medicine, CB #7070, Chapel Hill, NC 27599-7070.
E-mail address: charles_ebert@med.unc.edu

also extends into the pediatric realm, leaving a significant deficit in the understanding of pediatric sinonasal disease.[3]

Pediatric rhinosinusitis remains one of the most common diseases of childhood. Upper respiratory tract infections represent the most significant predisposing factor, with children averaging 6 to 8 infections annually. Of these infections, 0.5% to 5% progress to acute rhinosinusitis with an unknown percentage progressing to CRS.[3] Recent estimates indicate that patients diagnosed with CRS account for nearly 6 million pediatrician visits annually, with a substantial proportion of these being referred to subspecialty practitioners.[2]

CLASSIFICATION OF CRS

Rhinosinusitis is a group of disorders characterized by concurrent inflammatory and infectious processes that affect the nasal passages and the contiguous paranasal sinuses.[4] Traditionally, symptom duration has dictated the rhinosinusitis classification schema as follows: acute (>4 weeks), subacute (4–12 weeks), and chronic (more than 12 weeks, with or without acute exacerbations).

Acute rhinosinusitis may be further subdivided by symptom pattern into:

- Acute bacterial rhinosinusitis, characterized by symptoms lasting 10 or more days beyond the onset of upper respiratory symptoms or symptomatic worsening within 10 days after initial improvement, termed double-worsening
- Acute viral rhinosinusitis.

When there are 4 or more episodes of acute bacterial rhinosinusitis per year without persistent intervening symptoms, the term recurrent acute rhinosinusitis is applied.[5] Despite the ease and clinical applicability of the temporal scheme, classifications intended to guide clinical research have been described and include:

- Infectious etiology
- Complications
- Inflammatory markers
- Radiographic findings
- Endoscopic findings.

These systems of increased complexity allow for further patient subclassification and comparison of treatment modalities, which is of particular importance in the CRS population.

Clinical Diagnosis of Chronic Rhinosinusitis

CRS, as previously defined, is an inflammatory condition of the nasal passages and paranasal sinuses lasting 12 weeks or longer.[4] This heterogeneous and multifactorial disease process is clinically characterized by purulent drainage, polyps, and polypoid mucosa consistent with inflammation. Although nasal endoscopy is recommended and may reveal mucosal abnormalities of the middle meatus or sphenoethmoid recess, visual confirmation of these findings is not a required criterion. The diagnosis remains clinical, owing to the multitude of health care professionals caring for these patients.[2] The clinical diagnosis in children is often more challenging, with radiographic studies reserved for those being considered for surgery, rather than for diagnostic purposes.[6] In children, recurrent cough is a consistent sign and symptom of rhinosinusitis, and there is evidence to suggest that rhinosinusitis is an independent risk factor for the development of recurrent cough with wheezing.[7] Moreover, the diagnosis of CRS is rarely made in isolation and common comorbidities may include asthma, allergy, dental disease, polyposis, cystic fibrosis, and immunodefi-ciency syndromes.[2]

Detailed Classification of Chronic Rhinosinusitis

The heterogeneity of CRS has made classification challenging, and numerous schemes have been developed to further divide patients into more detailed groups.

One such scheme proposed by Meltzer divided rhinosinusitis into 4 categories[8]:

1. Acute presumed bacterial rhinosinusitis
2. CRS without polyps
3. CRS with polyps
4. Classic allergic fungal rhinosinusitis (AFS).

An alternative classification scheme proposed by Chan and Kuhn (F.A. Kuhn FA, MD, Savannah, GA, personal communication, 2009) divides CRS into 2 large cate-gories based on the type of inflammatory response.[4]

1. Noneosinophilic chronic rhinosinusitis (NECRS)
2. Eosinophilic chronic rhinosinusitis (ECRS).

NECRS is marked by neutrophilic inflammation and T-helper (Th)-1 cell predomi-nance. Pathologic subtypes of this designation include:

- Mechanical obstruction
- Chronic bacterial sinusitis without mucin or tissue eosinophilia
- Cystic fibrosis
- Primary ciliary dyskinesia
- Noneosinophilic rhinosinusitis with nasal polyps.

The latter example has recently been described by Borish,[9] who reported that non-eosinophilic polyps tend to display more profound glandular hypertrophy, fibrosis, and mononuclear and mast cell infiltrates than eosinophilic counterparts.

ECRS is marked by eosinophilic inflammation in the setting of Th-2 and interleukin-5 predominance, and is extremely difficult to control. It is hypothesized that some external trigger activates and upregulates these pathways in the setting of a genetic predisposition toward the characteristic eosinophilic response. Pathologic subtypes of ECRS include:

- Aspirin-sensitive asthma with nasal polyps
- AFS
- AFS without fungus
- *Staphylococcus aureus*–induced superantigen rhinosinusitis
- Chronic gram-negative rhinosinusitis with nasal polyps
- Eosinophilic CRS of unknown etiology.

FUNGAL SINUSITIS

There are 4 distinct types of fungal sinusitis with varying clinical presentations and physical examination findings:

1. Acute fulminant invasive fungal sinusitis
2. Chronic indolent invasive fungal sinusitis
3. Mycetoma or fungus ball sinusitis
4. AFS.

Invasive sinusitis is often a life-threatening condition that uniformly requires surgical debridement and aggressive antifungal therapy. The subtypes are distinguished from each other based on the course of onset and the populations affected.

Acute fulminant invasive fungal sinusitis is a life-threatening condition that is rapidly progressive and affects immunocompromised patients.

Chronic indolent invasive fungal sinusitis generally affects the immunocompetent population, and is marked by fungal invasion into the sinonasal mucosa.

Mycetoma or fungus ball sinusitis is characterized by noninvasive, fungal proliferation and expansion within a sinus in a nonatopic, immunocompetent patient, and can be definitively treated by debridement.

AFS represents the final type of allergic sinusitis and is the topic of the remainder of this discussion.[10]

ALLERGIC FUNGAL SINUSITIS

AFS is a distinct subtype of eosinophilic CRS marked by[10,11]:

- Type I hypersensitivity (by history, skin tests, or serology)
- Nasal polyposis
- Characteristic computed tomography findings (**Fig. 1**)
- Eosinophilic mucus (**Fig. 2**)
- Presence of fungal elements of the tissue removed during surgery without evidence of fungal tissue invasion (**Fig. 3**).

This entity was first recognized by Millar and colleagues,[12] who reported histopathologic similarities between materials obtained from the maxillary sinuses of 5 patients and pathologically diagnosed specimens of allergic bronchopulmonary aspergillosis. These findings were further described by Katzenstein and colleagues[13] who, following a retrospective review of 113 consecutive cases, identified 7 patients with a newly recognized form of chronic sinusitis termed allergic *Aspergillus* sinusitis. These patients were mostly young adults with a history of asthma and nasal polyposis. Radiographic findings revealed opacification of multiple sinuses. Histopathologic analysis of tissue resected from the paranasal sinuses demonstrated distinct mucinous material containing eosinophils, Charcot-Leyden crystals, and fungal hyphae (**Fig. 4**). This mucinous material was likened to the mucoid impaction seen

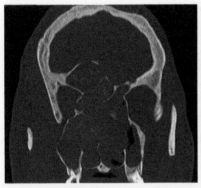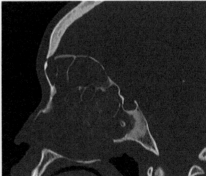

Fig. 1. Coronal and sagittal noncontrasted computed tomography maxillofacial scans from a pediatric patient with documented allergic fungal sinusitis. There is opacification of the bilateral paranasal sinuses with characteristic bony expansion and erosion.

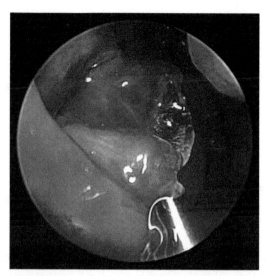

Fig. 2. Endonasal endoscopic view of allergic mucin within the paranasal sinuses of a pediatric patient with documented allergic fungal sinusitis.

in bronchopulmonary aspergillosis and shared similar histopathologic features, prompting the aforementioned terminology and providing evidence to support a pathophysiologic relationship between the 2 entities.[13] Bent and Kuhn[11] ultimately developed the diagnostic criteria for AFS in 1994 (**Box 1**). Numerous efforts have been made to modify the criteria for AFS, to clarify some inconsistencies in the clinical characteristics of cases.[14] However, the Bent-Kuhn criteria have remained the most widely accepted diagnostic method.

Further investigation into this distinct entity revealed a myriad of other dematiaceous fungi resulting in similar clinical manifestations. To avoid confusion, a change in terminology was made to the clinical term allergic fungal sinusitis.[14] In a recent study by (Melroy and colleagues, unpublished data, 2009) of 723 positive fungal cultures in 231 patients, the most common encountered genera in AFS were *Aspergillus*. However, other histologically similar dematiaceous fungi such as *Curvularia*, *Penicillium*, *Alternaria*, *Bipolaris*, and *Fusarium* have also been implicated. These data

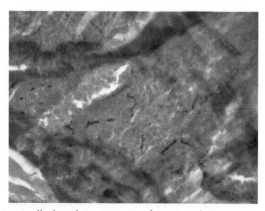

Fig. 3. Fungal elements displayed on a smear of paranasal sinus contents using Grocott's methenamine silver (GMS) stain.

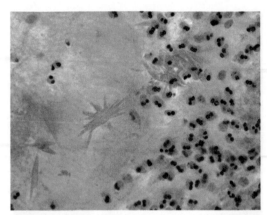

Fig. 4. Charcot-Leyden crystal displayed on a hematoxylin and eosin stain of allergic mucin.

suggest that the incidence of isolated fungal genera is likely related to the species distribution in the local environment, and that more than one fungal genera have a role in the disease process.

Epidemiology of Allergic Fungal Sinusitis

There are scant epidemiologic data on AFS in general, and even fewer in children. Nevertheless, AFS accounts for 7% to 12% of patients with chronic rhinosinusitis who undergo sinus surgery in the United States.[15,16] In addition, there appears to be a clear geographic pattern of distribution focused in temperate climates. Specifically, an increased incidence in the southern United States and the Mississippi Basin likely represents the influence of climatic factors on the fungal milieu.[17]

AFS is most common among adolescents and young adults: the mean age at diagnosis is 21.9 years. Although reports differ on the male-to-female (M/F) ratio of AFS, the ratio is relatively equal when accounting for the different age distributions of disease between the genders.[18] For example, McClay and colleagues[19] reviewed 151 patients with ages ranging from 5 to 75 years and found nearly a 1:1 M/F ratio. However, there may be an age-related difference in the M/F ratio when comparing children and adults. A review of children with AFS at University of Texas Southwestern revealed a distinct male predominance, with a 2.1:1 M/F ratio and an average age at diagnosis of 13 years.[18] Conversely, the adult population showed a female predominance, with an M/F ratio of 1:1.4 and an average age at diagnosis of 36 years.[18] One

---

Box 1
Diagnostic criteria for AFS

Type I hypersensitivity confirmed by history, skin testing, or serology

Characteristic computed tomography findings

Nasal polyposis

Histologic evidence of eosinophilic mucus without evidence of fungal invasion into sinus tissue

Positive fungal stain of sinus contents

Data from Bent JP, Kuhn FA. Diagnosis of allergic fungal sinusitis. Otolaryngol Head Neck Surg 1994;111(5):580–8.

other series of children with AFS also reported an M/F ratio of 1.5:1 with a mean age at diagnosis of 13.6 years.

There is scant data to indicate whether ethnicity portends any significant risk for developing AFS. However, at our institution, we have found a clear racial predominance: African Americans represent the vast majority of our patients, outnumbering all other races combined by a ratio of 4:1. Whether this trend is generalizable to the entire population of AFS patients remains unknown.

Diagnosis of Allergic Fungal Sinusitis

The etiologic basis of AFS is the abnormally robust immunologic response elicited by an allergy to ubiquitous fungal species. Therefore, it is not surprising that the criteria defining this disease include documented atopy and the presence of fungus (see **Box 1**). Minor diagnostic criteria also exist, and include the concurrent presence of:

- Asthma
- Charcot-Leyden crystals
- Eosinophilia
- Unilaterality of disease
- Evidence of osseous erosion
- Positive sinonasal fungal culture.

A review of 178 pediatric and adult patients diagnosed with AFS found that the average time to diagnosis from the initial visit was 11 months, with patients undergoing an average of 2.4 surgeries before diagnosis. Moreover, the earliest documented clinical feature was most frequently a computed tomography finding (5.15 months), and the latest criterion was a positive fungal smear (8.63 months). While characteristic computed tomography findings were often the earliest documented signs of disease in patients with AFS, 65% of patients did not display these findings at any point during the course of their disease (Melroy and colleagues, unpublished data, 2009).

Radiographic findings

Characteristic radiographic findings are clearly important for diagnosis and planning of surgical treatment. Computed tomography plays a key role in diagnosis in this patient population. Findings invariably include multiple opacified sinuses and a combination of osseous expansion and/or erosion. AFS displays significantly more osseous expansion and thinning of the bony confines of the sinonasal cavities than other forms of CRS, with 56% of cases presenting with radiographic evidence of skull-base erosion or intraorbital extension. By contrast, bony erosion/expansion was noticed in only 5% of other causes of CRS.[20] In children asymmetric disease predominates, with 70% of pediatric patients presenting with unilateral disease, compared with only 37% of adults.[19] Despite this increased propensity toward unilaterality, pediatric patients display comparable incidences of osseous erosion, especially of the intracranial anterior cranial fossa and orbit.[18]

Initial clinical diagnosis

The initial diagnosis of AFS is largely clinical and will likely be broadly termed CRS. This holds especially true for the pediatric population, where diagnostic radiographic studies may be less frequently used to minimize radiation exposure and are typically reserved for only those patients in whom surgical intervention is planned.[3] A detailed history coupled with a complete examination is necessary to elucidate the diagnosis. Concurrent comorbidities such as asthma and atopy must be elicited to reach an appropriate presumptive diagnosis. Atopy is a hallmark of the disease, with nearly 66% of patients reporting a history of allergic rhinitis (AR) and about 90% of patients demonstrating elevated specific immunoglobulin E (IgE) to 1 or more fungal antigens.[18] Furthermore, in a study by Manning and Holman,[21] roughly 50% of AFS patients were noted to have asthma.

Symptomatically, most children with AFS typically present with:

- Nasal airway obstruction
- Nasal discharge (at times purulent)
- Loss of smell/taste
- Headaches.

However, the presentation of AFS is children may be quite subtle.[19] The onset of AFS is typically a protracted, indolent process. Children report a slow onset of nasal airway obstruction and production of large, dark-colored nasal debris. Because of this gradual onset and progression, patients may develop facial dysmorphia with proptosis and/or telecanthus.[19,22–24] If pain is a presenting symptom, it generally indicates a concomitant bacterial infection.[18]

Endoscopy is the best method to adequately assess the nasal cavities. However, in children this may be neither feasible nor well tolerated. Therefore, a comprehensive history, noninvasive physical examination, and radiographic imaging are paramount. If endoscopy is tolerated, the examiner should interrogate the bilateral nasal cavities for evidence of allergic mucin, polypoid edema, or polyposis. Findings that include any of these in a patient with atopy necessitate further inquiry into the possibility of AFS. Although history and findings of physical examination are crucial, the definitive diagnosis of AFS relies on a combination of factors including histopathologic findings. Therefore, although one may be highly suspicious, the definitive diagnosis of AFS cannot be made until after surgical intervention.[25]

Management of Allergic Fungal Sinusitis

The treatment of AFS is both medical and surgical. With increasing awareness of the pathogenesis of the disease and its relationship with the eosinophilic inflammatory cascade, a paradigm shift has led to medical therapies aimed at suppressing inflammation rather than eradicating fungal pathogens. In addition, as with other forms of sinusitis, medical therapy is not simply an initial treatment whose failure results in surgery, but rather a concurrent and adjuvant measure given to enhance the effects of surgical intervention and increase the symptom-free interval.

Functional endoscopic sinus surgery is the intervention of choice in this patient population, as nearly all cases of AFS will require some form of surgical management. Management should focus on tissue preservation to maintain sinonasal mucociliary clearance and relief of mechanical obstruction. Clearance of the sinus contents is also paramount and typically yields substantial amounts of thick allergic mucin and/or fungal debris, which should be sent for histopathologic review for the presence of fungal elements and eosinophils. Retention of cells filled with allergic mucin appears to be a risk factor for early recurrence, and every effort should be made to safely minimize residual disease (Videos 1 and 2).[26] Meticulous preoperative planning and intraoperative care must be taken in these patients, as osseous expansion and erosion often distorts the normal sinonasal anatomy and obliterates bony barriers, thus placing adjacent structures at an increased risk of iatrogenic injury. Image guidance is critical for orientation and anatomic confirmation (see **Fig. 1**).

Pearls & Pitfalls: It should be noted that normal anatomic surgical landmarks may be altered because of the expansive nature of allergic fungal disease.

The goals of surgical management for primary and recurrent disease remain the same and include removal of mechanical obstruction, clearance of sinus contents, and creation of adequate outflow tracts while maintaining the functional capacity of the lining mucosa.

Surgery, while representing an important arm in the treatment of AFS, does not obviate the need for adjuvant medial therapy.[11] The pathophysiology of AFS and diagnostic criteria clearly indicate that it is not simply the presence of fungus but also the patient's response to this allergen that define the disease. Systemic steroids decrease the inflammatory response including sinonasal mucosal edema and polyp formation, and are typically used in an initial burst preoperatively and with a taper in the postoperative period.

Pearls & Pitfalls: A course of systemic corticosteroids preoperatively can significantly reduce inflammation, improving both patient symptoms and endoscopic visualization at the time of surgery.

Serial examinations guide the need for continued systemic therapy. In the pediatric population, early efforts are made to transition from a systemic regimen to intranasal topical steroid therapy. The importance of adjuvant medical therapy was clearly displayed by Kupferberg and colleagues[10] in their retrospective review of 26 pediatric and adult patients undergoing functional endoscopic sinus surgery for AFS. Using a novel endoscopic staging system, the success of various postoperative medication regimens were compared (**Table 1**). The results indicated that a significantly higher number of patients in the steroid-treatment group were maintained in stages 0 and I compared with patients in other groups who did not receive steroids. Moreover, once patients progressed to stage II or III disease it was unlikely that medical management could reverse the process, and repeat surgical management was universally necessary. These findings demonstrate the need for long-term suppressive therapy and serial endoscopic evaluations in postoperative AFS patients.[11] At the authors' institution, children who have completed the taper of oral corticosteroid therapy are transitioned to topical steroid treatment, typically with budesonide (0.5 mg) in 1 L of isotonic buffered saline. Patients irrigate, if possible, with 120 mL per nostril 2 times per day.

A wide range of other medical therapies may be used in children with AFS to target the intense eosinophilic response that results in polypoid inflammation. Immunotherapy with specific attention to the fungal-specific antigens is thought to decrease recurrence rates after surgery when combined with other medical treatments.[27] In addition, leukotriene

Table 1	
Kupferberg, Bent, Kuhn novel endoscopic grading system	
Stage	**Criteria**
0	No evidence of disease
I	Edematous mucosa/allergic mucin
II	Polypoid mucosa/allergic mucin
III	Polyps and fungal debris

Data from Kupferberg SB, Bent JP, Kuhn FA. Prognosis for allergic fungal sinusitis. Otolaryngol Head Neck Surg 1997;117:35–41.

receptor antagonists, monoclonal antibody selectively binding IgE, macrolide antibiotics, and steroid-impregnated antibiotic gels may have a place in the long-term management of the disease process, although data are lacking.[14] Some investigators have postulated that decreasing the fungal antigen load in the sinonasal cavities with either systemic or topical antifungal agents may be useful. However, these data have not demonstrated efficacy in controlling AFS.[28] In addition, it should be noted that neither surgical nor medical management is curative: every patient has the potential for recurrence, and therefore requires long-term follow-up and continuous management.

Future Directions for Allergic Fungal Sinusitis

To date, there continues to be some controversy regarding the diagnostic criteria because of temporal variations in the clinical features required to make the diagnosis of AFS. In lieu of systemic medical therapy, which entails known side effects, long-term treatment of AFS is being transitioned to topical therapies. Topical application of steroids, antibiotics, and/or antifungals via nebulized formulations or mixed-in irrigants have shown some promise anecdotally. However, there are no data currently demonstrating efficacies of these therapies. As our understanding of the pathophysiology of AFS deepens, particularly from a genetic standpoint, immunomodulation will likely be a mainstay of long-term medical management. Nevertheless, surgical intervention will continue to be an essential part of the overall treatment plan of the child with AFS. For this reason, it is imperative to integrate all of the tools in our armamentarium, both medical and surgical, to provide children with the greatest possibility of long-term control. Unfortunately, the exact proportions of medical or surgical management that should be used are not yet fully understood.[18]

SUMMARY

CRS in the pediatric population remains an area of great importance because of its high prevalence and the diversity of disease presentations. An understanding of the classification schema is critical to the appropriate management of each disease subtype. The most useful clinical delineation is between NECRS, characterized by upregulation of the Th-1 pathway, and ECRS, with an enhanced Th-2 response. AFS is a refractory subtype of ECRS, defined by an intense inflammatory response to fungal antigens that are ubiquitous in the environment. Although the pathogenic mechanisms that create this condition are largely unknown, early diagnosis during childhood is often possible through a comprehensive understanding of the risk factors of this disease and thorough history and physical examination. Clinically, this is useful in guiding the decision to pursue computed tomography scanning and medical and surgical interventions that could potentially provide earlier symptomatic relief.

From a surgical standpoint, the goals of therapy are to remove the physical obstruction of the sinus outflow tracts, debride polyps and debris that are filling the sinuses, and maintain the patency of the sinuses to restore that mucociliary function of the uninvolved sinonasal mucosa. In doing so, great care must be taken to avoid causing iatrogenic damage to the structures surrounding the sinonasal airspaces, particularly because of the remarkable anatomic deformities associated with this condition. Image guidance is a helpful tool in this regard, and should be universally used during these procedures.

Medical therapies remain a useful adjuvant to surgical intervention. Evidence indicates that oral and topical corticosteroids may be effectively used to control the underlying inflammatory process. Because of the risks associated with steroid use in children, sustained systemic courses should be avoided, and early transition to topical regimens is advocated because of their lower systemic bioavailability. As more research reveals the underlying pathogenic mechanisms of AFS, there will likely be a shift toward immunomodulation of the robust Th-2 response that is present in this disease process.

REFERENCES

1. Anand VK. Epidemiology and economic impact of rhinosinusitis. Ann Otol Rhinol Laryngol Suppl 2004;193:3–5.
2. Benninger MS, Ferguson BJ, Hadley JA, et al. Adult chronic rhinosinusitis: definitions, diagnosis, epidemiology, and pathophysiology. Otolaryngol Head Neck Surg 2003;129(Suppl 3):S1–32.
3. Lusk R. Pediatric chronic rhinosinusitis. Curr Opin Otolaryngol Head Neck Surg 2006;14:393–6.
4. Chan Y, Kuhn FA. An update on the classifications, diagnosis, and treatment of rhinosinusitis. Curr Opin Otolaryngol Head Neck Surg 2009;17:204–8.
5. Rosenfeld RM, Andes D, Bhattacharyya N, et al. Clinical practice guidelines: adult sinusitis. Otolaryngol Head Neck Surg 2007;137(Suppl):S1–31.
6. Ramadan HH. Pediatric sinusitis: update. J Otolaryngol 2005;34(Suppl 1):S14–7.
7. Sherril DL, Guerra S, Cristina MM, et al. The relation of rhinitis to recurrent cough and wheezing: a longitudinal study. Respir Med 2005;99:1377–85.
8. Meltzer EO, Hamilos DL, Hadley JA, et al. Rhinosinusitis: establishing definitions for clinical research and patient care. Otolaryngol Head Neck Surg 2004; 131(Suppl):S1–62.
9. Borish L. Allergic rhinitis: systemic inflammation and implications for management. J Allergy Clin Immunol 2003;112:1021–31.
10. Kupferberg SB, Bent JP, Kuhn FA. Prognosis for allergic fungal sinusitis. Otolaryngol Head Neck Surg 1997;117:35–41.
11. Bent JP, Kuhn FA. Diagnosis of allergic fungal sinusitis. Otolaryngol Head Neck Surg 1994;111(5):580–8.
12. Millar JW, Johnston A, Lamb D. Allergic aspergillosis of the maxillary sinuses [abstract]. Thorax 1981;36:710.
13. Katzenstein AA, Sale SR, Greenberger PA. Allergic *Aspergillus* sinusitis: a newly recognized form of sinusitis. J Allergy Clin Immunol 1983;72:89–93.
14. Ryan MW, Marple BF. Allergic fungal sinusitis: diagnosis and management. Curr Opin Otolaryngol Head Neck Surg 2007;15:18–22.
15. Ence BK, Gourley DS, Jorgensen NL, et al. Allergic fungal sinusitis. Am J Rhinol 1990;4(5):169–78.
16. Granville L, Chirala M, Cernoch P, et al. Fungal sinusitis: histologic spectrum and correlation with culture. Hum Pathol 2004;35:474–81.
17. Ferguson BJ, Barnes L, Bernstein JM, et al. Geographic variation in allergic fungal rhinosinusitis. Otolaryngol Clin North Am 2000;33(2):441–9.
18. McClay JE, Meyers AD. Allergic fungal sinusitis. Emedicine article. Available at: http://emedicine.medscape.com/article/834401. Accessed August 14, 2011.
19. McClay JE, Marple BF, Kapadia L, et al. Clinical presentation of allergic fungal sinusitis in children. Laryngoscope 2002;112(3):565–9.
20. Ghegan MD, Lee FS, Schlosser RJ. Incidence of skull base and orbital erosion in allergic fungal rhinosinusitis (AFRS) and non-AFRS. Otolaryngol Head Neck Surg 2006;134:592–5.
21. Manning SC, Holman M. Further evidence for allergic pathophysiology in allergic fungal sinusitis. Laryngoscope 1998;108(10):1485–96.

22. Marple BF. Allergic fungal rhinosinusitis: current theories and management strategies. Laryngoscope 2001;111:1006–19.
23. Gupta AK, Bansal S, Gupta A, et al. Is fungal infestation of paranasal sinuses more aggressive in pediatric population? Int J Pediatr Otorhinolaryngol 2005; 70:603–8.
24. Manning SC, Vuitch F, Weinberg AG, et al. Allergic aspergillosis: a newly recognized form of sinusitis in the pediatric population. Laryngoscope 1989;99:681–5.
25. Ryan MW. Allergic fungal rhinosinusitis. Otolaryngol Clin North Am 2011;44: 697–710.
26. Marple BF, Mabry RL. Allergic fungal sinusitis: learning from our failures. Am J Rhinol 2000;14:223–6.
27. Folker RJ, Marple BF, Mabry RL, et al. Treatment of allergic fungal sinusitis: a comparison trial of postoperative immunotherapy with specific fungal antigens. Laryngoscope 1998;108:1623–7.
28. Kuhn FA, Javer AR. Allergic fungal sinusitis: a four year follow-up. Am J Rhinol 2000;14:149–56.

Multisystem Disease and Pediatric Laryngotracheal Reconstruction

Jeremy D. Meier, MD[a], David R. White, MD[b],*

KEYWORDS

- Subglottic stenosis • Laryngotracheal reconstruction • Multisystem disease

KEY POINTS

- Laryngotracheal stenosis can be caused or further aggravated by numerous systemic diseases.
- A multidisciplinary approach is critical when evaluating and managing children with laryngotracheal stenosis and underlying systemic disease.
- Surgical outcomes of laryngotracheal reconstruction can be adversely affected when underlying systemic disease is not properly addressed.

Laryngotracheal reconstruction (LTR) in the pediatric patient requires a highly skilled and experienced multidisciplinary team. Rarely a child presents for LTR with isolated subglottic stenosis (SGS). Often these patients have multiple medical comorbidities either directly contributing to the underlying airway disease or affecting perioperative management. Understanding the relationship of coexisting systemic processes in the pediatric patient with an airway disorder is critical, because the consequences of poorly managed airway reconstruction can be devastating. The assistance of multiple subspecialties, including otolaryngology, anesthesia, pediatric surgery, pulmonology, gastroenterology, intensive care, medicine, and genetics, as well as medical support personnel in nursing, speech therapy, and social service expertise, are essential for optimal outcomes.[1]

MULTISYSTEM DISEASE IN THE CAUSE OF SGS

Pediatric airway reconstruction is performed for congenital or acquired laryngotracheal stenosis. Most SGS is acquired. Infection, autoimmune disease, or massive

---

The authors have nothing to disclose.

[a] Division of Otolaryngology – Head and Neck Surgery, Department of Surgery, University of Utah, 50 North Medical Drive, Room 3C120 SOM, Salt Lake City, UT 84132, USA; [b] Pediatric Otolaryngology, Department of Otolaryngology – Head and Neck Surgery, Medical University of South Carolina, 135 Rutledge Avenue, Suite 1130, MSC 550, Charleston, SC 29425, USA
* Corresponding author.
E-mail address: whitedr@musc.edu

polytrauma may directly cause acquired SGS or tracheal stenosis with pathologic foci inflicting damage in the airway.

In the early 1900s, the predominant cause for acquired SGS was trauma or infectious diseases such as tuberculosis, syphilis, and diphtheria. With the advent of antibiotics, stenosis resulting from infectious causes significantly decreased.

The practice of long-term intubation in neonates requiring mechanical ventilation was introduced in 1965.[2] This practice led to an increased incidence of SGS. Improved techniques for managing neonatal ventilation have reduced the impact of airway injury caused by intubation.[3,4] Despite these improvements, the predominant risk factor for SGS remains endotracheal intubation.[5] The endotracheal tube size, length of intubation, tube movement while intubated, traumatic intubation, and presence of infection or gastroesophageal reflux disease (GERD) all contribute to SGS formation in the intubated patient.[6]

Prematurity is consistently associated with acquired SGS.[7] Treating SGS in the premature neonate presents many unique challenges. Along with a stenotic airway, the premature infant often has compromised lung function with bronchopulmonary dysplasia, neurologic delay, and poor nutrition (**Fig. 1**).

PEARLS & PITFALLS: The premature patient is the prime example of the challenges encountered in performing LTR in a patient with multisystem disease.

Laryngeal surgery, external neck trauma, burns, or caustic ingestions may also cause SGS. Although rare in the pediatric patient, SGS may develop from systemic autoimmune processes such as Wegener granulomatosis, relapsing polychondritis, and sarcoidosis. Management in these patients initially focuses on treating the underlying disease process. LTR is then considered only after the autoimmune disease is well controlled.

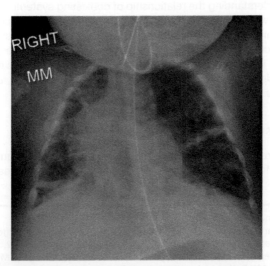

Fig. 1. Chest radiograph of premature infant with long-segment congenital tracheal stenosis secondary to complete tracheal rings. Image shows area of tracheal stenosis below the endotracheal tube and evidence of bronchopulmonary dysplasia. Additional comorbidities included chronic renal failure, necrotizing enterocolitis, and sepsis. The patient eventually underwent successful slide tracheoplasty once the underlying comorbidities were stabilized.

Congenital SGS currently accounts for only 5% of patients with SGS. Congenital SGS occurs in children without any prior intubations or other identifiable cause. The stenosis is attributed to an abnormally shaped cricoid cartilage or incomplete recanalization of the subglottis and is divided histologically into membranous and cartilaginous forms.[8] Children with Down syndrome are at greater risk of congenital SGS. Congenital tracheal stenosis, although rare, is frequently caused by a complete tracheal ring. Tracheal rings are often associated with a pulmonary vascular sling or intracardiac defects.

MULTISYSTEM DISEASE IN THE TREATMENT OF SGS
Severe SGS

Treatment options for SGS have increased greatly in the past 40 years. Before the introduction of airway reconstruction in the early 1970s,[9] tracheotomy was the primary long-term treatment of severe SGS. A tracheotomy tube completely bypasses the stenosis, avoiding more potentially invasive treatments of the diseased airway. This option is now most commonly used as a temporizing measure in patients not medically fit for extensive airway reconstruction. Patients with significant cardiopulmonary disease or other comorbidities, who would not tolerate a long general anesthetic, are tracheotomized to provide a secure and stable airway. Diseases known to affect the surgical outcome after laryngotracheoplasty, such as diabetes, upper airway infections, and gastroesophageal reflux, are medically treated and definitive airway reconstruction delayed until these patients are adequately managed.

Mild SGS

Patients with mild stenosis (grade I or mild grade II) may often be observed without any need for surgical intervention.[1] In patients with multisystem disease, decisions regarding management options ultimately necessitate a discussion weighing the risks versus benefits of intervention. Patients with intermittent crouplike symptoms that are exacerbated by upper respiratory tract infections can often be followed conservatively with surveillance endoscopy to ensure that the airway is growing with the child. An active, otherwise healthy child may be more symptomatic with mild-moderate SGS than a neurologically delayed or bed-bound child. Children with limited physical activity and functional abilities may be safer with a tracheotomy or close observation. The goals of any airway reconstruction in these children must be clearly defined by both the caregiver and the surgeon.

Laryngotracheal Stenosis

Laryngotracheal stenosis can be managed through open (transcervical) or endoscopic approaches. Advanced instrumentation and improved techniques have expanded the capabilities of endoscopic interventions in treating SGS in recent years. The endoscopic procedures prevent neck incisions and avoid many of the potential complications associated with open approaches. Balloon dilators, CO_2 lasers, powered microdebriders, and endoscopically placed costochondral grafts have all been used.[10–15] In the patient with multisystem disease, endoscopic operations provide potentially quicker and less invasive options that may be better tolerated.

Moderate to Severe SGS

Open transcervical approaches are the standard of care in the definitive treatment of moderate to severe SGS. These operations include airway expansion with interpositional cartilage grafts (eg, laryngotracheoplasty with anterior and posterior costochondral grafts) or segmental resection with primary anastomosis (eg, cricotracheal resection). Experienced surgical, anesthesia, and critical care personnel are essential because of the high acuity of these operations. Single-stage laryngotracheoplasty with interpositional cartilage grafts requires stenting via endotracheal intubation for several days. Postoperative pulmonary complications that accompany endotracheal intubation, such as atelectasis, consolidation, and pneumonia, are common. Prophylactic antibiotics are recommended to prevent infections at the site of reconstruction.

> PEARLS & PITFALLS: *Wound infections in the reconstructed airway can impair healing, destroy grafts, and contribute to the potentially deadly complication of airway dehiscence at the site of reconstruction.*

Voice and Swallowing Difficulties

Voice and swallowing difficulties are expected in the immediate perioperative period. Many patients with laryngotracheal stenosis have long-standing voice complaints secondary to prolonged endotracheal tube trauma to the vocal folds. After reconstruction, voice problems are often exacerbated in the expanded airway. Temporary dysphagia and aspiration may occur immediately after surgery but resolve in most cases within a short period of time. Speech language-pathology therapists are helpful in the long-term management of voice and swallowing mechanisms after airway reconstruction.

SPECIFIC MULTISYSTEM DISEASES AND LTR

The remainder of this article focuses on specific systems associated with laryngotracheal stenosis and reconstruction outcomes. These multisystem conditions must be addressed when determining management algorithms.

PULMONARY SYSTEM DISEASE

Children undergoing LTR frequently have compromised pulmonary function at baseline. Many of these children were premature and present with a history of chronic lung disease. Poor lung function necessitating long-term mechanical ventilation and endotracheal intubation often instigate the child's stenosis. A single-stage reconstruction typically requires a sedated and mechanically ventilated patient for several days, placing a patient with chronic lung disease at high risk of postoperative pulmonary complications. Aggressive pulmonary toilet and strict attention to ventilatory management are paramount to avoid atelectasis, mucus plugging, and pneumonia. Many children presenting for LTR have multilevel airway disease. In addition to subglottic or tracheal stenosis, distal airway conditions such as tracheobronchomalacia, or more proximal disorders in the supraglottis, such as laryngomalacia, may complicate the postoperative recovery.

One series examining complications after pediatric LTR found 6 cases of respiratory syncytial virus (RSV) bronchiolitis in 82 cases of single-stage LTR or CTR.[16] Major risk factors for RSV infection include prematurity, chronic lung disease, major congenital heart defects, pulmonary hypertension, immunodeficiency, or cystic fibrosis. Most children presenting for airway reconstruction have at least 1 of these risk factors. The investigators in this series recommend strict hygiene precautions to prevent nosocomial RSV infections and even suggest avoiding LTR procedures during peak RSV season.

CARDIOVASCULAR SYSTEM DISEASE

Children with congenital cardiac disease may be at increased risk of developing SGS because of recurrent and/or prolonged intubations required when treating the heart disease.[17] In addition, tracheal injury from intubation trauma coinciding with perioperative hypoperfusion during cardiopulmonary bypass in congenital cardiac patients may be more severe than typical intubation trauma.[18] With the exception of congenital tracheal stenosis, which is generally repaired at the time of the repair of cardiac defects, children with congenital heart disease and laryngotracheal stenosis may require delaying the reconstruction until the cardiac defects have been addressed. Despite the unique anesthetic and medical challenges that accompany these patients, children with congenital heart disease and laryngotracheal stenosis can undergo successful airway reconstruction. Pereira and colleagues[18] were able to achieve satisfactory airway outcomes after LTR in 7 of 8 patients with congenital heart disease.

Infants with congenital heart disease are also at higher risk of accompanying airway abnormalities. An association of anterior glottic web (**Fig. 2**) with DiGeorge or velocardiofacial syndrome (chromosome 22q11.2 deletion) has been identified.[19] These children often have the conotruncal heart defects present in velocardiofacial syndrome. Complete tracheal rings have also been associated with cardiovascular anomalies such as vascular sling[20] and other congenital cardiac defects.[21] These patients typically present with progressively worsening noisy breathing often described as a biphasic washing-machine sound.[21] As the child grows, the fixed diameter at the cartilaginous ring limits adequate expansion of the airway lumen. Slide tracheoplasty is usually the preferred procedure to correct complete rings, and can often be performed at the same time as the cardiovascular anomaly repair.

GASTROINTESTINAL SYSTEM DISEASE

Swallowing problems are frequently present in patients undergoing LTR. Many of these children have complex medical conditions requiring prolonged mechanical ventilation or neonatal intensive care requirements that prevent traditional oral

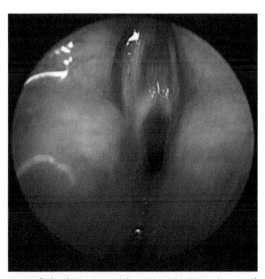

Fig. 2. Endoscopic view of the larynx reveals a pinpoint opening at the glottis caused by a laryngeal web. Laryngeal webs are frequently associated with velocardiofacial syndrome (chromosome 22q11.2 deletion) with accompanying conotruncal heart defects. The cardiac anomalies must be addressed when planning reconstruction for a stenotic airway such as the one depicted here.

alimentation. Oral aversion and other feeding difficulties frequently arise.[22] Before reconstruction, patients with airway stenosis may have difficulty maintaining adequate nutritional status primarily from oral means simply because of increased requirements related to protecting and maintaining the compromised airway. **Fig. 2** shows the preoperative and postoperative endoscopic views of an infant's subglottis after anterior and posterior costochondral cartilage grafts. The increased energy required to maintain an adequate airway while feeding affected the child's ability to sustain adequate nutrition. Significant volume loss of the posterior graft was noted and thought to be secondary to the patient's poor nutrition status before reconstruction. Transient dysphagia is expected after LTR.[23–25] However, Andreoli and colleagues[26] recently showed that most patients maintain their baseline feeding status after LTR.

Little and colleagues[27] showed GERD to be a pathogenic factor in the formation of SGS in a canine model. Children with SGS have been shown to have a high incidence of associated GERD.[6] In addition to contributing to the cause of SGS, GERD has been shown to affect management outcomes in SGS. Aggressively treating GERD before endoscopic intervention for SGS significantly improved outcomes.[28] Gray and colleagues[24] showed that uncontrolled GERD increased the risk of failure after LTR. Perioperative treatment of GERD is recommended in all patients undergoing LTR.

Eosinophilic esophagitis has been implicated as a complicating factor in the development of SGS.[29,30] This inflammatory disorder typically presents with recurrent emesis, regurgitation, feeding difficulties, or food impaction, and is characterized by infiltration of the esophageal epithelium with eosinophils.[30] In a series by White and colleagues[31] evaluating outcomes after cricotracheal resection, all 3 patients with eosinophilic esophagitis who underwent cricotracheal resection had an initial decannulation failure. Although the cohort was not large enough to be included in the multivariable analysis, a Fisher exact test showed significantly worse outcomes in these patients. The full impact of eosinophilic esophagitis in LTR is not understood. However, identifying and treating these patients before airway reconstruction helps to achieve optimal outcomes.

IMMUNE SYSTEM DISORDERS

Although uncommon in the pediatric population, autoimmune disorders such as Wegener granulomatosis and inflammatory diseases such as relapsing polychondritis can create significant laryngotracheal stenosis. Before any airway reconstruction can be considered in these children, the disease must be well controlled medically.

Treatment of Wegener granulomatosis typically includes corticosteroids and/or cyclophosphamide. A recent small series showed some success adding rituximab into the treatment regimen of children with Wegener granulomatosis and multilevel airway disease.[32] Airway interventions begin with endoscopic dilation and steroid injection, with tracheostomy insertion when needed (**Fig. 3**). The literature is too sparse to predict success rates regarding LTR in children with Wegener granulomatosis.

Relapsing polychondritis is a rare multisystem disease with recurrent inflammation and progressive destruction of cartilage and connective tissue. Auricular, nasal, or laryngotracheal cartilage is frequently affected. Nonerosive inflammatory arthritis, ocular inflammation, or vestibulocochlear lesions may also present. Obstructive airway symptoms occur from inflammatory swelling during the active phase (**Fig. 4**), cartilage destruction causing dynamic collapse, or fibrous tissue formation causing cicatricial contraction in the later stages.[33] Management begins with corticosteroids, although success has been reported with dapsone and immunosuppressive agents such as azathioprine and cyclophosphamide.[34] Because multilevel airway disease is common,

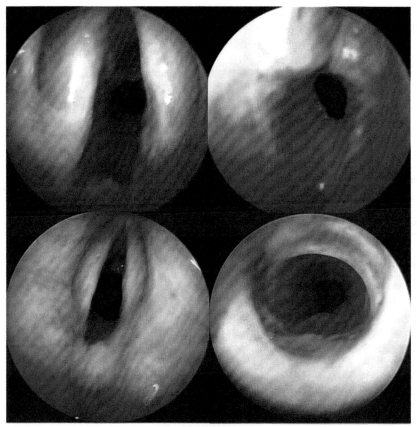

Fig. 3. Endoscopic views of subglottis in patient with Wegener granulomatosis. Upper panels show stenotic airway with active disease. Lower panels show improved airway after balloon dilation. LTR is deferred in patients with Wegener granulomatosis until maximal medical therapy and less invasive surgical options such as balloon dilation have been exhausted.

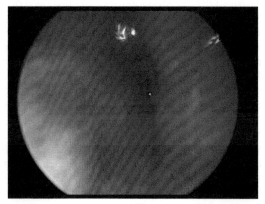

Fig. 4. Near-complete SGS in a patient with relapsing polychondritis. Despite the severe stenosis, LTR is usually deferred in these patients and children with this disease are often tracheotomy dependent.

LTR is rarely performed. Tracheostomy, balloon dilation, or airway stenting are usually attempted before considering a formal reconstruction. The literature only contains small case series or anecdotal reports of patients (usually adults) undergoing LTR for relapsing polychondritis.[34–36]

SUMMARY

Excellent surgical technique is only 1 side of the equation when performing airway reconstruction in the pediatric population. Children presenting for LTR usually have multiple comorbidities and disease processes affecting many other systems within the body. Adequately managing this multisystem disorder is essential to obtain good outcomes.

ACKNOWLEDGMENTS

Dr White is a consultant for Medtronic, Inc. and Gyrus ACMI; neither of these relationships are related to this article.

REFERENCES

1. Cotton RT. Management of subglottic stenosis. Otolaryngol Clin North Am 2000; 33(1):111–30.
2. McDonald IH, Stocks JG. Prolonged nasotracheal intubation: a review of its development in a pediatric hospital. Br J Anaesth 1965;37:161–73.
3. Choi SS, Zalzal GH. Changing trends in neonatal subglottic stenosis. Otolaryngol Head Neck Surg 2000;122:61–3.
4. Walner DL, Lowen MS, Kimura RE. Neonatal subglottic stenosis – incidence and trends. Laryngoscope 2001;111:48–51.
5. Bailey M, Hoeve H, Monnier P. Paediatric laryngotracheal stenosis: a consensus paper from three European centres. Eur Arch Otorhinolaryngol 2003;260:118–23.
6. Walner DL, Stern Y, Gerber ME, et al. Gastroesophageal reflux in patients with subglottic stenosis. Arch Otolaryngol Head Neck Surg 1998;124:551–5.
7. Silva OP. Factors influencing acquired upper airway obstruction in newborn infants receiving assisted ventilation because of respiratory failure: an overview. J Perinatol 1996;16:272–5.
8. Rutter MJ, Yellon RF, Cotton RT. Management and prevention of subglottic stenosis in infants and children. In: Bluestone CD, Stool SE, Alper CM, et al, editors. Pediatric otolaryngology. 4th edition. Philadelphia: Saunders; 2003. p. 1519–42.
9. Fearon B, Cotton RT. Surgical correction of subglottic stenosis of the larynx, preliminary report of an experimental surgical technique. Ann Otol Rhinol Laryngol 1972;81:508–31.
10. Mirabile L, Serio PP, Baggi RR, et al. Endoscopic anterior cricoid split and balloon dilation in pediatric subglottic stenosis. Int J Pediatr Otorhinolaryngol 2010;74: 1409–14.
11. Durden F, Sobol SE. Balloon laryngoplasty as a primary treatment for subglottic stenosis. Arch Otolaryngol Head Neck Surg 2007;133(8):772–5.
12. Lando T, April MM, Ward RF. Minimally invasive techniques in laryngotracheal reconstruction. Otolaryngol Clin North Am 2008;41:935–46.
13. Kirse DJ. Use of the microdebrider in pediatric endoscopic airway surgery. Curr Opin Otolaryngol Head Neck Surg 2009;17(6):477–82.
14. Rees CJ, Tridico TI, Kirse DJ. Expanding applications for the microdebrider in pediatric endoscopic airway surgery. Otolaryngol Head Neck Surg 2005;133(4):509–13.

15. Inglis AF, Perkins JA, Manning SC, et al. Endoscopic posterior cricoid split and rib grafting in 10 children. Laryngoscope 2003;113:2004–9.
16. Ludemann JP, Hughes CA, Noah Z, et al. Complications of pediatric laryngotracheal reconstruction: prevention strategies. Ann Otol Rhinol Laryngol 1999;108: 1019–26.
17. Khariwala SS, Lee WT, Koltai PJ. Laryngotracheal consequences of pediatric cardiac surgery. Arch Otolaryngol Head Neck Surg 2005;131:336–9.
18. Pereira KD, Mitchell RB, Younis RT, et al. Subglottic stenosis complication cardiac surgery in children. Chest 1997;111:1769–72.
19. Miyamoto RC, Cotton RT, Rope AF. Association of anterior glottic webs with velocardiofacial syndrome (chromosome 22q11.2 deletion). Otolaryngol Head Neck Surg 2004;130(4):415–7.
20. Sailer R, Zimmermann T, Böwing B, et al. Pulmonary artery sling associated with tracheobronchial malformations. Arch Otolaryngol Head Neck Surg 1992;118(8): 864–7.
21. Rutter MJ, Cotton RT, Azizkhan RG, et al. Slide tracheoplasty for the management of complete tracheal rings. J Pediatr Surg 2003;38(6):928–34.
22. Willging JP. Benefit of feeding assessment before pediatric airway reconstruction. Laryngoscope 2000;110:825–34.
23. Smith M, Mortelliti A, Cotton R, et al. Phonation and swallowing considerations in pediatric laryngotracheal reconstruction. Ann Otol Rhinol Laryngol 1992;101:731–8.
24. Gray S, Miller R, Myer CD, et al. Adjunctive measures for successful laryngotracheal reconstruction. Ann Otol Rhinol Laryngol 1987;96:509–13.
25. Zalzal G. Rib cartilage grafts for the treatment of posterior glottic and subglottic stenosis in children. Ann Otol Rhinol Laryngol 1988;97:506–11.
26. Andreoli SM, Nguyen SA, White DR. Feeding status after pediatric laryngotracheal reconstruction. Otolaryngol Head Neck Surg 2010;143:210–3.
27. Little FB, Koufman JA, Kohut RI, et al. Effect of gastric acid on the pathogenesis of subglottic stenosis. Ann Otol Rhinol Laryngol 1985;94:516–9.
28. Halstead LA. Gastroesophageal reflux: a critical factor in pediatric subglottic stenosis. Otolaryngol Head Neck Surg 1999;120:683–8.
29. Hartnick C, Liu JH, Cotton RT, et al. Subglottic stenosis complicated by allergic esophagitis: case report. Ann Otol Rhinol Laryngol 2002;111:57–60.
30. Dauer EH, Ponikau JU, Smyrk TC, et al. Airway manifestations of pediatric eosinophilic esophagitis: a clinical and histopathologic report of an emerging association. Ann Otol Rhinol Laryngol 2006;115:507–17.
31. White DR, Cotton RT, Bean JA, et al. Pediatric cricotracheal resection: surgical outcomes and risk factor analysis. Arch Otolaryngol Head Neck Surg 2005;131: 896–9.
32. Eustaquio ME, Chan KH, Deterding RR. Multilevel airway involvement in children with Wegener's granulomatosis. Arch Otolaryngol Head Neck Surg 2011;137:480–5.
33. Sarodia BD, Dasgupta A, Mehta AC. Management of airway manifestations of relapsing polychondritis: case reports and review of literature. Chest 1999;116: 1669–75.
34. Spraggs PD, Tostevin PM, Howard DJ. Management of laryngotracheobronchial sequelae and complications of relapsing polychondritis. Laryngoscope 1997; 107:936–41.
35. Karaman E, Duman C, Cansiz H, et al. Laryngotracheal reconstruction at relapsing polychondritis. J Craniofac Surg 2010;21:211–2.
36. Cansiz H, Yilmaz S, Duman C. Relapsing polychondritis: a case with subglottic stenosis and laryngotracheal reconstruction. J Otolaryngol 2007;36:E82–4.

A Review of the Evaluation and Management of Velopharyngeal Insufficiency in Children

James M. Ruda, MD[a],*, Paul Krakovitz, MD[b], Austin S. Rose, MD[c]

KEYWORDS

- VPI • Pharyngoplasty • Perceptual speech analysis • Nasal endoscopy
- Videofluoroscopy

KEY POINTS

- Velopharyngeal insufficiency (VPI) is an uncommon problem that typically manifests in patients as hypernasal speech, increased nasal resonance, nasal regurgitation, and nasal emission during phonation.
- VPI can occur sporadically but most often coexists as a syndromic finding (also known as velocardiofacial syndrome, submucosal cleft palate) or following previous operative intervention such as after cleft palate repair or adenoidectomy.
- Evaluation of VPI is multidisciplinary and revolves around initial perceptual speech evaluation by a speech-language pathologist, which is often combined with instrumental testing for confirmation.
- Treatment of VPI often initially involves a course of speech therapy for about 3 to 6 months before consideration of operative intervention as well as following most operative interventions to correct learned maladaptive speech patterns. However, most children are referred to the otolaryngologist after receiving prolonged speech therapy for hypernasal speech that fails to improve despite intensive therapy.
- Instrumental testing typically allows the surgical approach to be tailored based on the velopharyngeal (VP) gap size, location, and pattern of VP closure (VPC) that can involve of a superior-based pharyngeal flap versus sphincter pharyngoplasty versus posterior wall augmentation versus double-apposing Furlow Z-plasty versus prosthetic obturation.
- Operative repair of VPI is often undertaken after age 3 or 4 years when the patient is more cooperative with instrumental testing, which allows confirmation of the diagnosis and cause of VPI. Often, the earlier VPI is repaired, the fewer long-term speech problems and need for therapy exist. Occasionally, secondary repair is required, and this is successful in most children.
- Individual operative approaches may be used solely or in combination for VPI repair depending on the results of instrumental testing and the clinician's experience.

Financial disclosures/conflict of interest: The authors have nothing to disclose.
 a Department of Otolaryngology-Head and Neck Surgery, University of North Carolina, 170 Manning Drive, Chapel Hill, NC 27599-7070, USA; b Pediatric Otolaryngology, Head and Neck Institute, Cleveland Clinic, 9500 Euclid Avenue/A71, Cleveland, OH 44195, USA; c Department of Otolaryngology-Head and Neck Surgery, University of North Carolina School of Medicine, CB #7070, Chapel Hill, NC 27599-7070, USA
* Corresponding author.
E-mail address: ruda@med.unc.edu

Otolaryngol Clin N Am 45 (2012) 653–669
doi:10.1016/j.otc.2012.03.005
0030-6665/12/$ – see front matter © 2012 Elsevier Inc. All rights reserved.

▶ VIDEO OF VIDEOFLUOROSCOPY FOR THE EVALUATION OF PALATAL FUNCTION DURING SPEECH ACCOMPANIES THIS ARTICLE AT http://www. Oto.theclinics.com.

VP FUNCTION

The soft palate is commonly referred to as the velopharynx (VP). It is attached anteriorly to the hard palate via the palatal aponeurosis and is composed of multiple structures and muscles acting in a concerted fashion to produce VPC. These muscles include the paired muscles of the levator veli palatini and (LVP) tensor veli palatini (TVP), musculus uvulae, superior constrictor, palatopharyngeus, and palatoglossus muscles. Contraction of the VP elevates and retracts it posterosuperiorly in conjunction with simultaneous contraction of the lateral and posterior pharyngeal walls that move medially and anteriorly about 10 mm, respectively. Closure occurs at the level of the VP isthmus, whose location varies among individuals. Within the isthmus, sphincteric contraction with subsequent apposition of all structures within the nasopharynx functions to produce VPC, and this is typically located along the inferior aspect of the adenoid bed. VPC is required during attempted phonation, deglutition, and sucking, and serves to prevent nasal regurgitation of fluids or solids that are normally delivered to the oropharynx (OP). In addition, it functions to channel exhaled airflow and pressure from the vocal tract to the articulators of the oral cavity (tongue, teeth, lips) for normal resonant speech production. Coupling and uncoupling of the oral and nasal cavities occurs through rapid opening and closing of the VP valve, which permits regulated entry of sound pressure and energy into either the nasal or oral cavities during phonation. VPC also allows oral pressure development of 5 to 7 mm Hg to produce oral plosives or fricatives by the articulators.

Speech Production

Within the English language, all phonemes with the exception of /m/, /n/, and /ng/ are produced with oral airflow that requires VPC to exclude nasopharyngeal airflow. The presence of airflow leaking into the nasopharynx during normal oral speech or swallowing creates hypernasal speech, as well as excess nasal resonance, regurgitation, and audible emission, which occurs when a VP gap of greater than 10 mm^2 is present during attempted VPC. Only the /m/, /n/, and /ng/ phonemes require an open nasopharyngeal portal/valve and nasal airflow to produce these sounds. Hyponasality is a reduction in nasal resonance during phonation, especially of nasal phonemes such as /m/, /n/, and /ng/. It typically results from either partial or complete blockage of the nasal cavity or nasopharynx from mucosal edema associated with viral upper respiratory infection (URI), hypertrophic tonsils/adenoids, allergic rhinitis, hypertrophic turbinates, or anatomic obstruction from a deviated nasal septum or choanal atresia.[1,2] Hyponasality can be referred to diminished nasal resonance that occurs during the height of a URI when nasal mucosal congestion and obstruction are maximal. However, hyponasality and hypernasality may coexist in the same patient and make diagnosis of VPI difficult if hyponasality masks the hypernasal speech component. Referral to an otolaryngologist is advisable if hyponasal or hypernasal speech exist.

VP Anatomy and Action

Anatomically, contraction of the LVP provides posterosuperior elevation of the VP.

- The LVP derives its origin from the petrous portion of the temporal bone and from the medial lamina of the eustachian tube (ET).

- It descends with the ET from the temporal bone through the foramen of Morgagni to the level of the soft palate.
- It is innervated from the pharyngeal plexus of cranial nerve (CN) X and possesses muscle fibers that are oriented in a transverse fashion at the level of the VP. The pharyngeal plexus is also innervated via minor contributions from CN IX and CN VII.
- At the level of the VP, LVP fibers interdigitate in the midline with the contralateral LVP to form the VP sling.
- Anteriorly, the TVP originates from the base of the medial pterygoid plate, sphenoid spine, and lateral cartilaginous hook of the ET, and is innervated by CN V.
- Its tendinous fibers hook around the hamulus to insert into the anterior fibrous palatal aponeurosis of the soft palate, anterior to the LVP muscle. Contraction of this muscle serves to tense and stabilize the soft palate. In addition, given its origin from the ET, contraction of the TVP functions to open and close the ET via a pumping action.
- The musculus uvulae is a paired muscle that arises from the tendinous palatal aponeurosis anterior to the LVP and courses dorsal to the LVP to insert into the mucosa of the uvula.[3] It functions to elevate the uvula as well as to shorten and add bulk to the VP to occlude the VP port during speech and deglutition.[4] Absence of this muscle, especially in children with occult cleft palates or neuromuscular dysfunction, often results in VPI.

VPC is also obtained with the use of the palatopharyngeus and superior constrictor muscles primarily, which are innervated by the pharyngeal plexus. The palatopharyngeus muscles serve to elevate the pharynx and larynx during bolus transmission from the oral cavity to the hypopharynx. They also function to narrow the oropharyngeal aperture during swallowing.[5] Contraction of the superior constrictor muscle produces anterior and medial displacement of the posterior and lateral pharyngeal wall during deglutition, at the level of the first cervical vertebra. Within the area of the VP isthmus, 20% of all individuals may show development of a discrete transverse muscular ridge, also known as the Passavant ridge, which is produced during superior constrictor muscle contraction. However, it is controversial whether the Passavant ridge participates in VPC or is even located within the VP isthmus.

CLASSIFICATION OF VP DISORDERS

Disorders of the VP have been classified and/or named according to the underlying pathologic mechanism suspected to cause VPI. Within the literature, the nomenclature, including VP incompetence, insufficiency, inadequacy, and dysfunction, have been described, but are confusing as result of terminology used interchangeably without distinction or respect to the pathologic mechanism. With regard to children, the cause of VPI is typically anatomic, iatrogenic, or neuromuscular. VPI can also be classified as resulting from structural, functional, mechanical, or dynamic palatal (neuromuscular) abnormalities.[6,7]

Neuromuscular Abnormalities

Historically, VP incompetence has typically denoted a structurally intact VP affected by an underlying neurologic or musculoskeletal injury such as neuromuscular incoordination. This condition may be associated with an acute neurologic injury (CVA), intracranial processes, palatal paralysis, or progressive neurologic deterioration of the pharyngeal plexus (Amyotrophic Lateral Sclerosis, Parkinson disease, cerebral palsy, Möbius syndrome, Down syndrome). Neural injury may result in asymmetric weakness of the velopharynx and constrictor muscle if unilateral, or symmetric weakness in more severe cases. This condition can be associated with gross hypotonia and dysarthria. In more severe cases, weakness of the recurrent laryngeal nerve may also occur, resulting in dysfunction of vocal fold mobility, and the inability to generate adequate subglottic pressure for development of speech. Protective and reflexive acts such as gagging and swallowing may be impaired depending on the nature and the level of the lesion. This impairment includes lesions at CNs IX, X, XI, or the cerebellum.[8] VP incompetence may also result from a primary muscular disorder, although this is less common. It can occur in disorders such as muscular dystrophy. The velum and superior constrictor muscles may show evidence of gross hypomobility or immobility during voluntary speech and swallowing that result in dyscoordination of sphincteric closure and flaccid dysarthria.

Structural Abnormalities

VPI has been used to describe a neurologically intact VP that is structurally or anatomically deficient with respect to either position, size, soft tissue volume, or all of these variables. Examples include iatrogenic causes, such as following hard palatal advancement or adenoidectomy. In addition, it can occur in association with short palate syndrome, hard and soft cleft palate, nasopharyngeal disproportion, and so forth. Similarly, VPI may be produced from mechanical obstruction impairing VP mobility during speech and swallowing. This condition can occur secondary to tonsillar hypertrophy or tethering of the velum resulting from tonsillectomy, pharyngoplasty, or pharyngeal flap surgery that scars and stiffens the velum. It may also result from a palatal fistula complicating palatoplasty repair that allows airflow to escape from the oral to the nasal cavities.[8]

Articulation Abnormalities

VPI may arise from the presence of compensatory misarticulation that persists long after surgical repair of the palate. As described by Dworkin and colleagues,[2] this includes greater use of nasals, glides, glottal stops, pharyngeal stops and fricatives, posterior nasal fricatives, and fewer stop plosives that constitute articulatory avoidance behaviors and linguapalatal valving constraints.[2,8] This condition can also manifest as facial grimacing and low speech volume that act to reduce nasal airflow during oral phoneme speech. Ultimately, this can impair speech intelligibility and is difficult to correct, even with intense speech therapy. Similarly, mislearned errors of articulation or dialectical influences may also masquerade as VPI in a neuromuscularly intact child.[2] Although rare, this can occur in an atmosphere in which a child is exposed to mispronounced/misarticulated speech that is subsequently learned and replicated, leading to faulty speech patterns and behaviors. In addition, phoneme-specific misarticulations can occur when nasal emission is present with fricatives and affricatives in the absence of any hypernasal resonance.[8] In these instances, there is typically not a role for surgical intervention but instead speech therapy may be more beneficial. Thus, work-up for VPI must consider multiple causes during the diagnostic process. To simplify the frequent use of incorrect terminology, the term VP dysfunction or inadequacy is now more commonly used to describe abnormal VPC.

VPI ASSESSMENT

The diagnosis of VPI is typically ascertained by[9]:

- Routine historical intake
- Physical examination

- Combination of perceptual speech, instrumental evaluation, and reliance on the trained ear.

The physical examination focuses on detailed inspection of the oral and nasal cavities with attention to the velar height, mobility, and symmetry, and palatine tonsil size, tongue mobility and symmetry, oral competence, palatal and uvular appearance, as well as the nasal mucosa, turbinates, septum, and so forth. As is frequently described, attention to the OP searching for signs of a submucosal cleft palate (bifid uvula, zona pellucida, posterior palatal notching), as well as any anatomic or neuromuscular abnormality, is frequently undertaken. However, physical examination always overlooks an occult cleft palate and thus other instrumental evaluation is needed to make this diagnosis.

In addition, inquiry about any prior surgical intervention within the oral cavity or pharynx is discussed with the patient/family and is corroborated with examination findings of postoperative sequelae. These findings could include the presence of a palatal fistula, scarring, or mechanical obstruction of the VP valve. In the absence of findings, a detailed history is elicited for any known syndrome or neurologic abnormalities that may exist.

Dynamic mobility of the velopharynx is also inspected with the sustained phonation of the vowels /e/ or /i/. During this phase of the evaluation, the clinician may also observe for oral competence and the patient's ability to manage secretions, while evaluating for nasal regurgitation and presence of a gag reflex.

Perceptual Speech Evaluation

After a thorough history and examination, perceptual speech analysis is performed in conjunction with a multidisciplinary team that includes a speech-language pathologist along with otolaryngologist or plastic surgeon. Frequently, the diagnosis of VPI has been suspected previously or entertained by the patient's family or primary care physician before referral to the otolaryngologist.

Diagnostically, perceptual analysis connotes the use of the evaluator's unaided senses, whereas instrumental includes all evaluations that involve some type of instrumentation.[10,11]

Perceptual analysis

Perceptual analysis, the gold standard of VPI evaluation, includes listening to the spontaneous or prompted production of specific pressure phonemes including plosives, fricatives, and affricatives while monitoring for misarticulations, hypernasal speech, nasal rustle, and facial grimacing. It may also use articulation measurement, equal-appearing interval scales, and global ratings to assess VPI.[12] Facial grimacing is a compensatory action used by the patient to narrow the external nares to decrease nasal air emission during non-nasal speech. Use of the dental mirror placed under the nares during vowel production, may also assist in determining the amount of visible nasal air emission as shown by fogging of the mirror.

Within the office setting, VPI screening for VP inadequacy can also be performed by having the patient count from 60 to 80 while listening for the presence of nasal emission and hypernasal speech. Repetition of characteristic phrases such as "pet the puppies," "pick the peppers," and "Kathy kissed the cat" are frequently used as test phrases. For these tasks, coordination with a speech-language pathologist who possesses dedicated training and interest in the area of VPI is critical given the acknowledged subjective nature of perceptual evaluation. At present, there is no standardized perceptual acoustic evaluation protocol that is uniformly used among all speech-language pathologists throughout the United States, other than the International Working Group recommendations that were developed in the 1990s. Perceptual analysis may be supplemented with the use of the Pittsburgh Weighted Speech Scale, which is used in many clinics to report the severity of VPI when attempting comparative analyses.[6]

Instrumental assessment

Instrumental assessment is complementary to perceptual analysis during the evaluation of VPI. It is performed with two-dimensional or three-dimensional technology that uses either video-nasal endoscopy or multiview videofluoroscopy in either the presence of the surgeon, radiologist, or speech-language pathologist. In many centers, evaluation of VPI may also use pressure-flow measurements to determine the size of the VP port associated with the patient's VPI. Video-nasal endoscopy allows direct visualization of both nasal passages and nasopharynx with inspection of all nasal structures as well as the adenoids, nasopharyngeal depth, and soft palate mobility and size. It optimally uses the largest pediatric flexible laryngoscope that the child's anatomy and cooperation will accommodate, which is passed through the middle meatus to the nasopharynx. Endoscopic images are displayed on an attached video monitor for real-time simultaneous viewing by the speech-language pathologist who is directing the patient during the phonetic evaluation. During evaluation, VPC is assessed during multiple maneuvers, such as simulated sucking through a straw, as well as testing of oral and nasal phoneme production of fricatives, affricatives, plosives, and so forth. The patient is usually instructed to repeat key phrases during the examination. Ultimately, this allows determination of the location of VPC while scrutinizing VP gap geometry and correlating this with adjacent nasopharyngeal landmarks. Simultaneously, it also allows critical assessment of the degree of mobility or hypomobility of all VP structures, which helps guide the preoperative surgical decision-making. Nasal endoscopy also allows assessment for an occult cleft palate during visualization of the nasopharyngeal surface of the velum. Should a midline dimpled concave contour, or seagull sign, be found in the normal central convex velum, an occult cleft, representing a musculus uvulae deficiency, should be entertained as a cause for the patient's VPI.

Videofluoroscopy in Evaluation of VPI

Multiview videofluoroscopy is a two-dimensional radiologic instrumental analysis that is frequently used in the evaluation of VPI. It uses serial radiographs that are oriented in a lateral, frontal, and base view to analyze the VP valve and assess closure. It is often preferentially used in younger children who are unlikely to cooperate for a nasoendoscopic examination. It involves instillation of barium transnasally to coat the soft palate as well as the posterior and lateral pharyngeal walls. Subsequently, serial images of VPC are acquired of the cervical vertebrae and the posterior pharyngeal wall and Passavant ridge. Limitations include oversimplification of VPC in 1 plane, underestimation of the anteroposterior pharyngeal dimension, and tendency to suggest VPC when midline unilateral or bilateral defects exist.[13,14] Given the speed at which VPC occurs compared with the speed at which serial radiography can occur, videofluoroscopy has been criticized for the potential to suggest VPI when normal VPC is present. Despite this, videofluoroscopy is often used in conjunction with nasal endoscopy when it is not possible to ascertain levator orientation and VPC using only endoscopic evaluation. At our institution, we always attempt awake versus asleep nasal endoscopy performed with light sedation if possible, for reasons previously stated.

See Video 1 for an example of a Televex study incorporating videofluoroscopy for the evaluation of palatal function during speech.

Cephalometrics

Cephalometric evaluation uses principles common to videofluoroscopy that involve serial radiographs from an X-ray source during sustained speech and at rest to study various anatomic relationships obtained from multiple views of the pharynx. These views include:

- Cranial base angle
- Nasopharyngeal depth
- Velar length
- Dimpling
- Gap
- Stretch.

These variables allow comparison of the velar dimpling location that relates to the most anterior insertion of the levator muscle into the soft palate, in addition to the diagnosis of platybasia and cervical spine abnormalities contributing to nasopharyngeal disproportion. With increased anterior insertion, velar stretch is inversely decreased (as seen in submucosal and occult cleft palates) with the production of a potential velar gap during phonation. Limitations include VPI evaluation performed via static two-dimensional imaging and the need for radiation exposure. However, it is reported to be greater than 90% predictive of the need for pharyngeal flap surgery, as well as reliable, quantifiable, and useful in the evaluation and treatment planning of children with velocardiofacial syndrome and isolated cleft palates.[15] However, it cannot predict the amount of VPC required by corrective pharyngeal surgery.

MRI

In the past 5 years, MRI evaluation of the VP has also been increasingly used to study VPI because it is noninvasive, not associated with radiation exposure, and possesses reproducible imaging quality. Its role in VPI evaluation is still largely academic given its prohibitive cost and frequent need for procedural sedation during evaluation of children.[1] Although touted as dynamic imaging, it conceptually uses static imaging during limited speech that is often nonconnected and is not performed during multiple speech contexts. It is arguably used to assess LVP mobility and function, as well as assessing LVP muscle size, distribution, and orientation/position in cases in which submucosal or occult clefting of the VP is suspected.[16,17] This is achieved by following the length of the LVP from origin to insertion in multiple planes, which allows visualization of the direction and final insertion location of its distal muscular fibers into the soft palate. Ultimately, it compares favorably with nasal endoscopy and videofluoroscopy as a complementary tool for the evaluation of VPI, but its mainstream use is hampered by its prohibitive cost.

Nasometry

Nasometry is an objective, indirect test that is used to measure nasal emission. It allows the reproducible calculation of a ratio between nasal and oral sound emissions, known as nasalance, which can be compared with normative values of means and standard deviations (SDs). Preoperative and postoperative nasometric scores may be compared with postoperative success, often defined as within 1 SD from the normative mean. However, nasometry does not allow the localization or quantification of VP gap size. Large gaps may produce less high-pressure airflow detected by the nasometer and thus have an artificially depressed nasometric score compared with a small VP gap.

During instrumental assessment, the velopharynx is assessed for its unique closure pattern, which has been previously classified as either coronal, sagittal, or circular (symmetric). As described previously, coronal closure of the velopharynx involves mobility of only the posterior OP wall and VP with little contribution from the lateral OP walls. Conversely, sagittal closure refers to the active muscular contraction of the lateral OP walls with minimal contribution from the posterior OP wall, soft palate, or uvula. Circular closure refers to involvement of all structures, including the posterior and lateral OP walls, soft palate, and uvula, which contract equally to close the VP port. Endoscopic evaluation assists in determining the exact contribution of each structure either symmetrically or asymmetrically in producing VPC. Although this form of evaluation is imperfect, the benefit pertains to the lack of radiation exposure to the child during videofluoroscopic evaluation. However, a limitation to this diagnostic modality is the amount of voluntary cooperation during successive testing that is required to assess the VP port endoscopically, the pattern of VPC, and degree of contribution from all VP musculature during VPC. In addition, obstructive adenoids and the obliquity of view may hinder ideal visualization of the VP port.[13,14]

At our institution, nasal endoscopic examination is occasionally accomplished in the operative setting under light sedation using nitrous oxide in the presence of the speech-language pathologist. Although suboptimal, it allows assessment of all aforementioned objectives while avoiding videofluoroscopy. Typically, evaluation under light sedation is performed in children less than 4 to 5 years of age, given the difficulty in performing endoscopic examination in this young age group. However, endoscopic assessment data often influence the decision regarding how to proceed surgically with either a pharyngoplasty versus pharyngeal flap based on the visualized closure pattern and recognized deficient or immobile segment of the velopharynx. In multiple studies, tailoring of the superior pharyngeal flap width and length to the VP gap and closure point is often accomplished and with high postoperative success. Limitations of endoscopic evaluation typically include obliquity and skewing of VP port image, parallax errors, wide-angle distortion, and variability between endoscope operators, scope technology, and the clinician's technique.

EVALUATION OF VPI

Global management of VPI must account for the comprehensive impact of all VP-related issues on the health of the children. Questions pertaining to obstructive sleep apnea (OSA), as well as chronic eustachian tube dysfunction (ETD) with altered auditory discrimination, require historical investigation and treatment. Before any surgical intervention, OSA is often evaluated by polysomnography if the history warrants, and is often later addressed with routine tonsillectomy/adenoidectomy, if needed, around 6 to 8 weeks before any planned pharyngoplasty or palatoplasty. If discovered, the presence of OSA may also influence the decision to perform a posterior pharyngeal flap versus a sphincteroplasty.[1] In 20% of children, OSA is reported to develop as a late complication following pharyngeal flap surgery and can warrant flap takedown or additional surgery for correction. Performing tonsillectomy and adenoidectomy 2 months before any definitive VPI surgery allows adequate soft tissue healing within the tonsillar fossa and nasopharynx as well as allowing ample time for postoperative scar tissue formation and maturation to occur. It may also improve ease of sphincter myomucosal flap placement and approximation or posterior pharyngeal wall augmentation within the VP isthmus, which may be affected by hypertrophic, uninvolved adenoid tissue. In addition, evaluation of the larynx is critical because children with VPI often attempt to overcome their incompetent VP mechanism with increased laryngeal and respiratory effort. This effort can result in potential development of muscle tension dysphonia and laryngeal abnormalities such as development of vocal nodules and mucosal edema.[2]

Pediatric Syndromes

VPI is a frequent characteristic common to numerous syndromes within the pediatric population. Often VPI may result from either the presence of a structurally deficient palate, also known as cleft palate, or a gross muscular hypotonia that is found in many children presenting with neurologic and musculoskeletal abnormalities. VPI may be a predominant feature of a syndrome or equally may coexist among a wide constellation of findings that are pathognomonic for the specific syndrome. Knowledge and recognition that VPI may occur in relation to multiple syndromes is critical during the initial diagnostic evaluation of a child with VPI. Numerous common childhood syndromes that the otolaryngologist is likely to encounter in clinical practice with the unifying finding of VPI are listed later.

Cleft palate

Overt cleft palate occurs in approximately 1 in 650 to 750 children born annually and is the most common cause of syndromic VPI. It can occur in children sporadically or within the larger context of Pierre-Robin sequence, Stickler syndrome, craniofacial microsomia, or Kabuki syndrome. VPI in children born with a cleft palate results from the physical presence of a hard or soft palate cleft that prohibits oronasal separation before surgical repair. After surgery, VPI occurs in 20% of patients secondarily to palatal scarring and stiffness. It may also result from a functional but short reconstructed velum versus a nonfunctional but structurally normal velum that results from LVP musculature disorientation. It may also arise from the development of a palatal fistula complication. Children in whom VPI results after palatoplasty may also represent velar insufficiency that arises from interval growth of the velum and increased nasopharyngeal depth relative to a short velum. This condition may relate to the phenomenon of the palatoplasty inhibiting the palatal stretch factor in up to 57% of children who gradually undergo adenoid involution during normal growth and maturation. Removing the adenoids at the time of palatoplasty is generally not performed secondary to the known reduced stretch factor in children with cleft palate. Should adenoidectomy ultimately be required, a limited cephalad adenoidectomy is often undertaken nearest the choanae, taking care to preserve the posterior inferior adenoid pad against which the velum contacts.[18,19] VPI following cleft palate repair thus depends on multiple factors such as type of cleft, age at surgical repair, surgical technique, and presence of adenoids, with children whose cleft palate is repaired earlier typically developing more normal speech patterns.[6] When to perform velopharyngoplasty among all children is debatable, although multiple studies by Abyholm and colleagues[20] showed the greatest chance for VPI resolution in children operated on before age 7 years.

Submucosal cleft palate

Submucosal cleft palate (SMCP) is an uncommon occurrence, with a prevalence of 1:1250 to 1:6000. As described by Calnan,[21] the diagnosis is rendered in the presence of 3 morphologic findings:

1. Bifid uvula
2. Absent posterior nasal spine and presence of hard palate clefting
3. Presence of a zona pellucida that represents separation of the LVP muscles in the midline.

However, in multiple publications, the classic Calnan[21] triad may only be present in 25% to 93% of children, with concordance of all 3 findings found in as few as 24% of patients.[22] It may also present with the typical findings of chronic ETD and middle ear effusion, hypernasal speech, and VPI. Up to 17% to 55% of patients with VPI may have SMCPs that can occur in association with syndromic malformations such as Down syndrome.[12,22] However, the severity of SMCPs ranges from asymptomatic in greater than 70% to 90% of individuals to severe symptomatic VPI and chronic ETD. Because so many patients with SMCPs are asymptomatic, it is often recognized that the incidence of this disorder is grossly underestimated.

It is difficult to diagnose SMCPs visually given that the causal malformation is hidden deep to intact mucosa in young children who are often not cooperative during the office oropharyngeal examination. An SMCP may be diagnosed at the time of routine repeat myringotomy and tube placement or during tonsillectomy/adenoidectomy when the palate is more easily visualized. Failure to consider or render this diagnosis during surgery in a child with SMCP can lead to the development of VPI. The presence of a bifid uvula at the time of surgery is often quoted to herald the presence of possible SMCP. An isolated bifid uvula is typically quoted to occur in 1% to 7% of children overall.[12,22] Postadenoidectomy VPI is typically attributed to marginal VPC that was present before surgery whereby veloadenoidal closure was the predominant mechanism for VPC. It is often thought that postadenoidectomy VPI results from the presence of an occult cleft palate or SMCP. After surgery, veloadenoidal closure is suddenly absent following adenoidectomy, thus eliminating the posterior contact point for the velum and rapidly transitioning to VP valve closure. About 25% of children with Down syndrome present with an SMCP that fails to improve with intense speech therapy and ultimately requires surgical intervention. Within this population, a short velum has been noted that contributes to palatal insufficiency as well as altered developmental oromotor functions. As reported by Andreassen and colleagues,[23–26] children with cleft palate, congenital palatal incompetence, SMCP, facial paralysis, Down syndrome, nasal regurgitation in infancy, anomalies to the upper cervical vertebrae and cranial base, and family history of VPI or cleft palate, should be considered high risk for postoperative VPI formation. Should VPI development after adenoidectomy, treatment typically involves a trial of speech therapy for 6 to 12 months before considering the need for secondary surgical repair.

Velocardiofacial syndrome

In the past 10 years, one of the most common syndromic causes of VPI in noncleft patients has been the recognition of the role of velocardiofacial syndrome (VCFS) in this population. VCFS was first described by Shprintzen[27] and primarily affects 1:2000 to 1:4000 individuals who carry a 3-megabase pair microdeletion in the region of chromosome 22q11 that is known as the DiGeorge critical region. More than 75% to 85% of patients with the VCFS phenotype carry this microdeletion anomaly. In others, interstitial deletions of chromosome 4q, unbalanced translocations of chromosome 22, and deletions in the short arm of chromosome 10p13/14 can occur.[28] It is commonly associated with DiGeorge syndrome, conotruncal anomaly face syndrome, as well as Cayler cardiofacial and autosomal dominant Opitz-G/BBB syndrome.[28] VCFS is associated with a multitude of classic features such as dysmorphic facies, conotruncal cardiac defects, hypocalcemic hypoparathyroidism, T-cell mediated immune deficiency, and palate abnormalities, as well as more than 300 different abnormalities. Within this syndrome, there is extreme variability of findings that are not addressed in detail in this article. There can also be alterations in learning, speech, and feeding, as well as psychiatric disorders. The disorder may arise sporadically or be inherited in an autosomal dominant fashion. It is most commonly detected with fluorescent in-situ hybridization probe analysis using the Tuple I and ARSA markers. With VPI, approximately 70% of VCFS children are affected as well as having feeding problems (40%–90%) and speech/language delay. Approximately 40% of patients with VCFS also develop chronic ETD, recurrent otitis media with effusion, and conductive hearing loss. VCFS has also frequently been associated with the development of anterior glottic webbing in neonates and children. It is also associated with laryngomalacia, bronchomalacia, vascular rings, and laryngeal webs.[29]

OTHER SYNDROMES ASSOCIATED WITH VPI
Muscular Dystrophy

Muscular dystrophy is a heritable syndrome that progressively affects skeletal muscles of the body either systemically or focally among muscle groups and produces muscle atrophy and wasting. The oculopharyngeal variety is known to affect the musculature of the upper head and neck including the pharyngeal muscles involved with swallowing. VPI is produced with involvement of the LVP or TVP muscles or pharyngeal constrictors muscles. There is no known cure or treatment of this disease. Surgical treatment of VPI is not generally performed given the poor prognosis and rapid deterioration.

Myasthenia Gravis

Similar to muscular dystrophy, myasthenia gravis is a disease that affects the skeletal muscles in an autoimmune fashion. Myasthenia gravis classically affects voluntary muscles whose function worsens with activity and improves with rest. This disease targets the acetylcholine receptor involved in neuromuscular signal transmission. Functions of the head and neck are typically impaired such as swallowing, phonation, and gaze fixation, with the production of hoarseness, diplopia, dysphonia, upper eyelid ptosis, and difficulty maintaining head stability.

Möbius Syndrome

Möbius syndrome is another uncommon heritable syndrome that can be associated with VPI. It is primarily an uncommon congenital neurologic disease affecting CNs VI and VII in most patients but also CNs VIII and V in a smaller percentage of patients. Should it affect CN V, weakness of the TVP can result in incompetence of the VP valve. VPI may also be caused by cerebral palsy, which is a nonprogressive motor disease in children that affects motor development and coordination. It can involve multiple types and exist in varying degrees of severity. Unlike the more common hypertonic, contracted spastic-type cerebral palsy, hypotonic cerebral palsy can present with gross motor weakness of the affected region of the body or affect the body systemically. VPI can result if the muscles of the head and neck are involved, especially the VP musculature.

   Like all other syndromic causes of VPI, treatment involves assessing the amount of VPC and closure pattern of the child and individually tailoring the surgical or nonsurgical intervention to each child's underlying cause.

TREATMENT OF VPI

Treatment of VPI is multifaceted and considerations during treatment planning must include[30]:

- Underlying suspected cause.
- VPC pattern.

- VP gap size and symmetry.
- Age of patient.
- Associated syndrome.
- Potential for the VPC pattern to evolve or worsen during the child's lifetime.
- Whether the underlying cause of the VPI represents a neuromuscular versus anatomic abnormality, because this strongly affects the overall surgical decision.
- Trial of targeted speech therapy for about 6 months to determine whether nonoperative treatment can improve function enough to avoid surgery. It can be successful in mild cases of VPI. However, in more severe cases of VPI, most patients require surgery and postoperative speech therapy. The latter is used to address either remnant hypernasal speech patterns or to correct misarticulations and maladaptive learned behaviors that were previously used to compensate for hypernasal speech.
- Impact of further anatomic growth of the child in regard to the nasopharyngeal port's geometry and size relative to the velum and pharyngeal walls. Growth of the child may contribute to the eventual recurrence of VPI despite initial surgical success.
- If the VPI was iatrogenically induced following adenoidectomy, in which case the problem relates only to an anatomic deficiency in tissue but suspected normal neuromuscular function, then simple supplementation of the posterior OP wall or narrowing of the VP isthmus may suffice to restore the VP valve closure. However, if multiple structures within the VP port are functionally weak or with restricted mobility, but are structurally normal, then the degree of correction may need to overcompensate for future functional deterioration. This correction is often accomplished with a pharyngeal flap or sphincter pharyngoplasty.

All of these factors must ultimately be considered before surgery, during the diagnostic evaluation process, to guide the choice of surgical intervention for each child who presents with VPI.[31,32] In most children, VPI treatment is planned after the age of 3 or 4 years, when a child's degree of cooperation permits instrumental testing and quality data to be obtained regarding VPC patterns and tissue needs.

Multiple Procedures to Lengthen the Velum

Historically, treatment of VPI secondary to a short palate after cleft palatoplasty has involved multiple procedures designed to lengthen the velum. Palatal setbacks or Furlow double-apposing Z-plasties have frequently been used to accomplish this purpose by borrowing mucoperiosteum from the adjacent hard palate to lengthen the velum and reposition the sagittally oriented LVP muscles. Typically, patients with less severe VPI with VP gaps less than 5 mm and a small active VP sphincter have been treated with the Furlow palatoplasty method. In some patients, Furlow Z-plasty can be combined with a pharyngeal flap or sphincter pharyngoplasty to correct their VPI.[31] Overall, Furlow pharyngoplasty is less likely to be associated with postoperative nasopharyngeal obstruction or OSA because it does not obstruct or narrow the nasopharyngeal lumen.[33]

Augmentation Pharyngoplasty

Augmentation pharyngoplasty has been used for treatment of VPI associated only with a small central VP gap of less than 3 to 4 mm within the VP valve. It is typically not used in patients who possess gaps within the lateral VP valve. Augmentation pharyngoplasty involves anterior displacement of the central posterior pharyngeal wall to restore or provide a contact point for the velum during VPC. Historically, augmentation pharyngoplasty of the nasopharynx has used multiple substances such as silicone, cartilage, collagen, Vaseline, rolled posterior pharyngeal wall, fat, fascia, paraffin, silicone, acellular dermis, polytetrafluoroethylene, and calcium hydroxylapatite (CAHA).[34–36] Substances are typically placed within the retropharyngeal space just deep to the superior constrictor muscle but superficial to the pharyngobasilar fascia. Although use of autologous tissue is well tolerated, it is often complicated by the risk of resorption, infection, extrusion, and need for multiple injections. In addition, visualization of aberrant vasculature in the retropharyngeal space is critical before dissection to avoid inadvertent carotid injury in syndromic patients with VCFS.

CAHA and Autologous Fat

Within the past 5 years, CAHA and autologous fat have been increasingly used to augment the posterior pharynx in children with mild VPI. As described by Brigger and colleagues[35] and Leuchter and colleagues,[36] it is often used for children with a small central VP gap, marginal VPC, or who have minimal touch closure of the velum against the adenoid tissue.[34–36] It is often avoided when a lateral VP gap exists given the inconsistency with obtaining postoperative VPC closure. It may be used in patients in whom a pharyngeal flap or pharyngoplasty is considered overly aggressive, such as in a child with minimal VPI or with a poor prognosis arising from other medical comorbidities. However, augmentation pharyngoplasty can also be used in children with intermittent hypernasal speech and mild nasalization. Approximately 2 to 4 mL of CAHA injected into the retropharyngeal space tends not to migrate after injection if placed properly. Injection into the wrong tissue plane can be problematic with either fat or CAHA. In most patients, VPI was corrected within most patients after 1 to 2 serial injections without need for additional nonaugmentative surgery. However, if required, any future surgical success was not compromised by the presence of CAHA or fat in the retropharyngeal space. With autologous fat injections, overinjecting by at least 30% to 50% is often required to offset the anticipated resorption that commonly occurs.[37] Overall, injection pharyngoplasty with CAHA or fat provides sufficient VPC in patients with central small VP gaps, such as in patients after adenoidectomy with postoperative VPI development.

Pharyngeal Flap Surgery

Pharyngeal flap surgery is one of the most common procedures undertaken in children with VPI that results from a syndromic versus nonsyndromic origin. Overall, it is quoted to be successful in patients with poor VPC resulting from hypotonia, poor posterior and lateral pharyngeal wall mobility, and those with coronal VPC patterns. It is commonly used in the VCFS patient population with great success. Pharyngeal flaps function by creating a permanent passive obturation of the nasopharynx using posterior pharyngeal wall muscle and mucosa that is joined to the posterior surface of the VP. It compensates for poor mobility of all VP structures by providing static obturation of the VP, leaving 2 lateral ports after surgery for nasal airflow. It simultaneously narrows the nasopharyngeal isthmus via primary closure of the pharyngeal donor defect, which medializes the pharyngeal walls when reapposed.[32] However, creation of lateral VP ports in 5% to 27% of patients may result in postoperative hyponasality from overobturation of the nasopharynx when VP ports are less than 25 mm^2. In addition, in 20% of patients, postoperative development of sleep apnea and nasopharyngeal obstruction may occur.[38] It may also be associated with postoperative lateral port stenosis.

In most patients, pharyngeal flaps are currently fashioned as superiorly based, with the flap width determined by the VP gap, mobility and length of the palate, level of

VPC, and closure pattern that was noted on nasal endoscopy. Flaps are typically inset symmetrically because previous attempts to skew pharyngeal flaps for asymmetric defects did not improve postoperative VPC or resolution of VPI. Although flaps can be designed or tailored to incorporate variable widths of posterior pharyngeal wall, often one-third to two-thirds of the pharyngeal wall are used to fully obturate the central VP port. Afterward, all raw surface area of the pharyngeal flap is lined with native nasopharyngeal mucosa to prevent the postoperative contraction and tubular formation that develops with exposed raw muscle. Failure to do so results in a variable contraction of the flap and suboptimal obturation of the nasopharyngeal isthmus with persistent VPI. After surgery, children are monitored for oxygen desaturations, snoring, hyponasal speech, and OSA. Should OSA develop after surgery, most children are observed in the short term and considered for continuous positive airway pressure, if tolerated, or possible flap takedown in the long term. Even after flap takedown, the results of pharyngeal flap surgery have been reported to be preserved. It is speculated that this occurs because the native velum still possesses the remnant posterior pharyngeal flap tissue that was lysed from its donor attachment site and still acts to add bulk to the velum during VPC. Failure to resolve VPI after surgery in children after pharyngeal flaps occurs in a reported 4% to 12% of patients who require additional surgery. Typically, most surgeons wait for a variable amount of time for flap and velar healing before committing to a revision pharyngeal flap surgery, if required. This surgery can involve a Z-plasty technique or division of the pharyngeal flap from the velum as well as consideration for a sphincter pharyngoplasty or possible Furlow Z-plasty, depending on the patient's anatomy.

PEARLS & PITFALLS: Children should be monitored closely for possible OSA following pharyngeal flap surgery.

Sphincter Pharyngoplasty

Like pharyngeal flap surgery, sphincter pharyngoplasty is another common velopharyngoplasty used to correct VPI in children. This pharyngoplasty technique provides dynamic muscle action and physiologic activity of the velum by creating a dynamic sphincter of variable diameter that preserves the flexibility of the velum.[39] Among some institutions across the country, it rivals the superior-based pharyngeal flap as the workhorse for VPI repair. Sphincter pharyngoplasty was originally proposed and later modified by Orticochea,[40] whose design is still frequently replicated even to this day. It involves bilateral lysis of the posterior palatopharyngeal muscle/ tonsillar arch inferiorly or along the midpoint of the muscular arch. Afterward, these flaps are rotated and anchored onto the posterior pharyngeal wall as superior as possible to rest in the VP isthmus. On anchoring both palatopharyngeal muscles to the pharyngeal wall and horizontally overlapping the opposing muscle bundles and suture approximating them, a sphincteric tightening of the pharynx is created. This process effectively medializes the lateral and posterior wall of the superior constrictor muscles to reduce the transverse diameter of the VP port. As reported by multiple investigators, it is also associated with minimal to no postoperative OSA development because the central VP port is not obstructed.[39] However, this technique relies on the presence of a mobile velum and normal levator orientation to produce anterior-posterior velar movement to close the VP valve. It can also be combined with a Furlow Z-plasty and secondary velopharyngoplasty for treatment of VPI with excellent results and minimal risks.[33] It can even be taken down and the sphincter readjusted via tightening the limbs of the palatopharyngeus stumps secondarily should VPI persist after initial pharyngoplasty.

SUMMARY

Evaluation and management of VPI is complex and broad. VPI may occur sporadically or present as either a landmark feature or a synchronous finding among others that innately define multiple syndromes. Evaluation of VPI is multidisciplinary and revolves around initial perceptual speech evaluation with the speech-language pathologist that is often combined with instrumental testing for confirmation. Instrumental testing typically allows the formulation of an optimal strategy for operative intervention based on the VP gap size, location, and pattern of VPC. This strategy often includes, superior-based pharyngeal flap versus sphincter pharyngoplasty versus posterior wall augmentation versus nonoperative management with speech therapy or artificial obturation.

The ideal intervention for each patient depends on multiple factors. Surgical obturation of the VP gap is successful in most patients but is fraught with multiple postoperative complications such as bleeding, OSA, persistent VPI, pain, and infection. Should postoperative failure occur following surgical intervention, various treatment options still exist and are frequently used. Understanding the intricacies and nuances of VPI evaluation and management is thus critical for the otolaryngologist given the likelihood of encountering a patient with VPI.

REFERENCES

1. Rowe MR, D'Antonio LL. Velopharyngeal dysfunction: evolving developments in evaluation. Curr Opin Otolaryngol Head Neck Surg 2005;13(6):366–70. Grade B.
2. Dworkin JP, Marunick MT, Krouse JH. Velopharyngeal dysfunction: speech characteristics, variable etiologies, evaluation techniques, and differential treatments. Lang Speech Hear Serv Sch 2004;35(4):333–52. Grade B.
3. Azzam NA, Kuehn DP. The morphology of musculus uvulae. Cleft Palate J 1977; 14(1):78–87. Grade B.
4. Pigott RW, Bensen JF, White FD. Nasendoscopy in the diagnosis of velopharyngeal incompetence. Plast Reconstr Surg 1969;43(2):141–7. Grade B.
5. van Aalst JA, Kolappa KK, Sadove M. MOC-PSSM CME article: nonsyndromic cleft palate. Plast Reconstr Surg 2008;121(Suppl 1):1–14. Grade B.
6. Rudnick EF, Sie KC. Velopharyngeal insufficiency: current concepts in diagnosis and management. Curr Opin Otolaryngol Head Neck Surg 2008;16(6):530–5. Grade B.
7. Conley SF, Gosain AK, Marks SM, et al. Identification and assessment of velopharyngeal inadequacy. Am J Otolaryngol 1997;18(1):38–46. Grade B.
8. Johns DF, Rohrich RJ, Awada M. Velopharyngeal incompetence: a guide for clinical evaluation. Plast Reconstr Surg 2003;112(7):1890–7 [quiz: 1898, 1982]. Grade B.
9. Willging JP. Velopharyngeal insufficiency. Curr Opin Otolaryngol Head Neck Surg 2003;11(6):452–5. Grade B.
10. Marsh JL. Velo-pharyngeal dysfunction: evaluation and management. Indian J Plast Surg 2009;42(Suppl):S129–36. Grade B.
11. Marsh JL. Management of velopharyngeal dysfunction: differential diagnosis for differential management [Erratum appears in: J Craniofac Surg 2003;14(6):936]. J Craniofac Surg 2003;14(5):621–8 [discussion: 629]. Grade B.
12. Gosain AK, Conley SF, Marks S, et al. Submucous cleft palate: diagnostic methods and outcomes of surgical treatment. Plast Reconstr Surg 1996;97(7): 1497–509. Grade B.
13. Pigott RW. An analysis of the strengths and weaknesses of endoscopic and radiological investigations of velopharyngeal incompetence based on a 20 year experience of simultaneous recording. Br J Plast Surg 2002;55(1):32–4. Grade B.

14. Pigott RW. Velopharyngeal (speech) disorder (VP(S)D) without overt cleft palate. Br J Plast Surg 1994;47(4):223–9. Grade B.

15. Veerapandiyan A, Blalock D, Ghosh S, et al. The role of cephalometry in assessing velopharyngeal dysfunction in velocardiofacial syndrome. Laryngoscope 2011;121(4):732–7. Grade B.

16. Shprintzen RJ, Marrinan E. Velopharyngeal insufficiency: diagnosis and management. Curr Opin Otolaryngol Head Neck Surg 2009;17(4):302–7. Grade B.

17. Perry JL, Kuehn DP. Magnetic resonance imaging and computer reconstruction of the velopharyngeal mechanism. J Craniofac Surg 2009;20(Suppl 2): 1739–46. Grade B.

18. Silver AL, Nimkin K, Ashland JE, et al. Cine magnetic resonance imaging with simultaneous audio to evaluate pediatric velopharyngeal insufficiency. Arch Otolaryngol Head Neck Surg 2011;137(3):258–63. Grade B.

19. Tweedie DJ, Skilbeck CJ, Wyatt ME, et al. Partial adenoidectomy by suction diathermy in children with cleft palate, to avoid velopharyngeal insufficiency. Int J Pediatr Otorhinolaryngol 2009;73(11):1594–7. Grade B.

20. Abyholm F, D'Antonio L, Davidson, et al. Pharyngeal flap and sphincterplasty for velopharyngeal insufficiency have equal outcome at 1 year postoperatively: results of a randomized trial. Cleft Palate Craniofac J 2005;42(5):501–11. Grade B.

21. Calnan J. Submucous cleft palate. Br J Plast Surg 1954;6(4):264–82. Grade B.

22. Reiter R, Brosch S, Wefel H, et al. The submucous cleft palate: diagnosis and therapy. Int J Pediatr Otorhinolaryngol 2011;75(1):85–8. Grade B.

23. Andreassen ML, Leeper HA, MacRae DL, et al. Aerodynamic, acoustic, and perceptual changes following adenoidectomy. Cleft Palate Craniofac J 1994; 31(4):263–70. Grade B.

24. Finkelstein Y, Berger G, Nachmani A, et al. The functional role of the adenoids in speech. Int J Pediatr Otorhinolaryngol 1996;34(1–2):61–74. Grade B.

25. Haapanen ML, Ignatius J, Rihkanen H, et al. Velopharyngeal insufficiency following palatine tonsillectomy. Eur Arch Otorhinolaryngol 1994;251(3):186–9. Grade B.

26. Saunders NC, Hartley BE, Sell D, et al. Velopharyngeal insufficiency following adenoidectomy. Clin Otolaryngol Allied Sci 2004;29(6):686–8. Grade B.

27. Shprintzen RJ, Goldberg RB, Lewin ML, et al. A new syndrome involving cleft palate, cardiac anomalies, typical facies, and learning disabilities: velo-cardio-facial syndrome. Cleft Palate J 1978;15(1):56–62. Grade B.

28. Cuneo BF. 22q11.2 deletion syndrome: DiGeorge, velocardiofacial, and conotruncal anomaly face syndromes. Curr Opin Pediatr 2001;13(5):465–72. Grade B.

29. Sell D. Issues in perceptual speech analysis in cleft palate and related disorders: a review. Int J Lang Commun Disord 2005;40(2):103–21. Grade B.

30. Armour A, Fischbach S, Klaiman P, et al. Does velopharyngeal closure pattern affect the success of pharyngeal flap pharyngoplasty? Plast Reconstr Surg 2005;115(1):45–52.

31. Witt PD, Marsh JL. Advances in assessing outcome of surgical repair of cleft lip and cleft palate. Plast Reconstr Surg 1997;100(7):1907–17. Grade B.

32. Swanson EW, Sullivan SR, Ridgway EB, et al. Speech outcomes following pharyngeal flap in patients with velocardiofacial syndrome. Plast Reconstr Surg 2011; 127(5):2045–53. Grade B.

33. Wójcicki P, Wójcicka K. Prospective evaluation of the outcome of velopharyngeal insufficiency therapy after pharyngeal flap, a sphincter pharyngoplasty, a double Z-plasty and simultaneous Orticochea and Furlow operations. J Plast Reconstr Aesthet Surg 2011;64(4):459–61. Grade B.

34. Lypka M, Bidros R, Rizvi M, et al. Posterior pharyngeal augmentation in the treatment of velopharyngeal insufficiency: a 40-year experience. Ann Plast Surg 2010; 65(1):48–51. Grade B.
35. Brigger MT, Ashland JE, Hartnick CJ. Injection pharyngoplasty with calcium hydroxylapatite for velopharyngeal insufficiency. Arch Otolaryngol Head Neck Surg 2010;136(7):666–70. Grade B.
36. Leuchter I, Schweizer V, Hohlfeld J, et al. Treatment of velopharyngeal insufficiency by autologous fat injection. Eur Arch Otorhinolaryngol 2010;267:977–83. Grade B.
37. Cantarella G, Mazzola RF, Mantovani M, et al. Treatment of velopharyngeal insufficiency by pharyngeal and velar fat injections. Otolaryngol Head Neck Surg 2011;145(3):401–3. Grade B.
38. Cole P, Banerji S, Hollier L, et al. Two hundred twenty-two consecutive pharyngeal flaps: an analysis of postoperative complications. J Oral Maxillofac Surg 2008;66: 745–8. Grade B.
39. Saint Raymond C, Bettega G, Deschaux C, et al. Sphincter pharyngoplasty as a treatment of velopharyngeal incompetence in young people: a prospective evaluation of effects on sleep structure and sleep respiratory disturbances. Chest 2004;125(3):864–71. Grade B.
40. Orticochea M. Construction of a dynamic muscle sphincter in cleft palates. Plast Reconstr Surg 1968;41(4):323–7. Grade B.

Recurrent Respiratory Papillomatosis

Naren N. Venkatesan, MD, Harold S. Pine, MD,
Michael P. Underbrink, MD*

KEYWORDS

- Papillomas • Papillomatosis • Aerodigestive tract • Human papillomavirus

KEY POINTS

- Recurrent respiratory papillomatosis (RRP) is a rare, benign disease with no known cure, affecting millions of children; incidence is increased with lower socioeconomic status.
- RRP is caused by infection of the upper aerodigestive tract with the human papillomavirus (HPV). More than 100 types of HPV have been identified; the low-risk HPV types 6 and 11 are responsible for RRP.
- Transmission of RRP typically occurs from mother to neonate. Passage through the birth canal is thought to be the initial transmission event, but infection may occur in utero.
- HPV vaccines have helped to provide protection from cervical cancer; however, their role in the prevention of RRP is undetermined.
- Clinical presentation of initial symptoms of RRP may be subtle, including hoarseness, dyspnea, chronic cough, or recurrent upper respiratory infections.
- RRP course ranges from aggressive with pulmonary involvement to isolated laryngeal disease with spontaneous remission.
- Current management focuses on surgical debulking of papillomatous lesions with or without concurrent adjuvant therapy.
- Common adjuvant therapies used currently include cidofovir and interferon (IFN).

⊙ VIDEO OF TECHNIQUE OF MICRODEBRIDER FOR REMOVAL OF PAPILLOMAS ACCOMPANIES THIS ARTICLE AT http://www.oto.theclinics.com/.

RRP is the term used to describe infection of the upper aerodigestive tract by human papilloma virus (HPV). Although papillomas may present anywhere along the tract, the larynx is the most common location.[1,2] RRP typically presents in a bimodal pattern during either adult life or early childhood. The latter presentation is marked by a more aggressive and recurring course, and therefore is commonly referred to

Department of Otolaryngology, University of Texas Medical Branch, 7.104 John Sealy Annex, 301 University Boulevard, Galveston, TX 77555-0521, USA
* Corresponding author.
E-mail address: mpunderb@utmb.edu

Otolaryngol Clin N Am 45 (2012) 671–694
doi:10.1016/j.otc.2012.03.006
0030-6665/12/$ – see front matter © 2012 Elsevier Inc. All rights reserved.
oto.theclinics.com

separately as juvenile RRP. Because of this unpredictable course, knowledge and management of RRP is essential to any otolaryngology practice.

INCIDENCE OF RRP

Transmission of juvenile RRP occurs from the mother to the child either in utero or at the time of birth. The increase in prevalence of HPV cervical infections in women has been mimicked by an increase in RRP. Although it is difficult to ascertain the incidence of RRP, it is estimated that juvenile RRP is present in 4.3 per 100,000 people in the United States.[3] As discussed later, the incidence of RRP has been greater in patients of lower socioeconomic status, another fact correlating with the increased incidence of HPV in this population. This belief was recently validated further by a pilot study of a large database of publically and privately insured patients in the United States. The study showed that the RRP incidence was higher in publically insured patients compared with privately insured patients by more than 150%: 3.21 versus 1.98 per 100,000, respectively.[4]

The Hospital for Sick Children in Toronto showed that nearly half of juvenile patients with RRP were below the poverty line for Canadian citizens.[5] This finding further reinforces the idea that patients of lower socioeconomic status are at increased risk. However, no correlation has been found between socioeconomic status and severity of the disease.[5]

ECONOMIC EFFECTS OF RRP

Currently, there is no cure for RRP and so treatment is directed at preventing upper airway compromise and improving vocal function while preserving laryngeal tissues. Because of the infectious and proliferative nature of RRP disease, affected patients are prone to frequent recurrences and multiple surgical treatments. This disease not only affects individual patients significantly but also places a large economic burden on their families and society in general. Typical pediatric patients require nearly 20 surgical procedures throughout their lifetimes, many of which occur early in the children's lives. During the initial years of the disease, a child is estimated to require slightly more than 4 surgeries per year.[6] Nearly 19% of children manifest a more aggressive course of the disease, requiring greater than 40 procedures in their lifetimes.[7] The average lifetime cost to treat 1 patient with RRP has been estimated at $60,000 to $470,000 in the United States.[4] On a national level, it is estimated that there are 15,000 surgical procedures performed every year in adults and children with RRP, with a total health care cost of nearly $150 million.[3]

RESEARCH INTO RRP

Although certain aspects of RRP continue to remain enigmatic, the disease's morbidity and significant economic burden are well established and underscore its clinical relevance. With any disease, some fundamental information regarding the epidemiology and virology provides a baseline for understanding. As a complex pathogen, the complete picture of the molecular mechanism of disease is still unclear; however, this aspect remains a key area of current research. Further, as a disease whose prevalence is growing, the transmission process as well as the role of recently introduced HPV vaccines is discussed. In addition, clinical manifestations and management of these patients continues to evolve with the advancement of new surgical technology and pharmaceutics.

Causes/Epidemiology of RRP

Through demonstration of papillomata on his arm, Ullman[8] first confirmed the presence of an infectious agent in laryngeal papillomas in 1923. RRP was then confirmed to contain HPV DNA in 1980. Further characterization and typing was done by

Gissman and colleagues[9] and Mounts and colleagues,[10] which confirmed the hypothesized role of HPV.

HPV is an icosahedral DNA capsid virus that is categorized based on genetic homology into greater than 180 identified genotypes, which correspond with different tissue preferences and clinical manifestations. HPV types 6 and 11 account for most cases of RRP. HPV-11 occurs most commonly (50%–100% of isolates)[9–14] and runs the most aggressive clinical course, followed by HPV-6. HPV types 16, 18, 31, and 33 have also been reported in RRP, albeit rarely.[15]

HPV types affecting the mucosal tracts can be broadly divided into high-risk and low-risk types based on their ability to cause malignant transformation of epithelial cells. High-risk types HPV-16 and HPV-18 are most commonly associated with cervical cancers as well as a subset of oropharyngeal carcinomas. HPV-6 and HPV-11 are considered low-risk types, not typically associated with malignancy, although transformation in RRP has been described. The rate of malignant transformation in RRP is less than 1%,[16] and has generally been reported in adults with other risk factors such as tobacco use or exposure to radiation but also in children with prolonged, extensive disease and distal spread.[17–19] The cause of transformation is thought by some investigators to follow a gradual molecular transformation. In one example, this involved integration of HPV-11 DNA into the host genome in malignant tissue samples and mutation of the p53 proto-oncogene.[18,20]

In their largest series of 9 patients, Reidy and colleagues[20] found HPV-11 to be present in all evaluable malignant samples, and RNA assays showed evidence of HPV integration in 3 of 7 sufficient samples. No evaluation of p53 status was performed in this study. In 5 sufficient samples from 7 patients with malignant transformation, Go and colleagues[21] agreed with the consistent expression of HPV-11 in malignancy, and found p53 expression to be variable, but was not able to show a progressive histologic appearance in serial samples. The palliative treatment for benign RRP is redirected when malignant transformation occurs, using conventional head and neck cancer oncological principles that supersede the original "tissue sparing" goals. Most squamous cell carcinomas (SCCA) arising with a history of RRP are well differentiated, and, when occurring in the lung, seem to have a refractory course.

The question has also been raised regarding the presence of HPV in the clinically disease-free larynx and respiratory tree.[17] Although ethical concerns make it difficult to explore this area in disease-free human subjects, a meta-analysis has shown that up to 10% of normal-appearing oral mucosa contained high-risk HPV.[22] Furthermore, normal-appearing adjacent mucosa or areas appearing to be well treated may show dormant HPV when tested for HPV DNA rather than for histologic changes, as shown by the finding of HPV DNA in macroscopically normal sites in patients with RRP at a rate of 61%.[23] This latent HPV DNA may then become reactivated and cause recurrence of papillomas. As with other viral pathogens, stress on the patient's immune system may also serve as the trigger for the virus replication. One recent study showed that children with RRP have reduced CD 4/CD 8 ratios and poor lymphocyte response to mitogen stimulation, implying that these children have inadequate cell-mediated immunity.[24] Thus, a deficient host immune system is likely another factor in the development of recurrent disease.

HPV Virology

The HPV is an icosahedral capsid DNA virus in the family Papovaviridae. It contains no envelope and has a double-stranded DNA genome containing approximately 8000 base pairs. HPV has a propensity for infecting epithelial cells. Although only select types are associated with RRP, more than 100 types of HPV have been identified, varying in the species they infect and the epithelial tissue they prefer. HPV infects stem cells within the basal layer of mucosa.

HPV genome
The HPV genome consists of 8 genes coding for E1, E2, E4, E5, E6, E7, L1, and L2. The L1 and L2 proteins are transcribed late in the viral life cycle and are responsible for producing the viral capsid. The E designation refers to genes that are transcribed early in the viral life cycle and are responsible for replication of the viral genome using host cellular machinery. These early genes also encode for potent oncoproteins that interact with many host cellular proteins and can cause transforming activities and disrupt cell growth and function. The most studied of these are the E6 and E7 proteins, which have been shown to prevent apoptosis and alter cell cycle function. They target the p53 and retinoblastoma tumor suppressor proteins, respectively. The tumor suppressor, p53, is an important cellular protein serving the important cellular functions of sensing and stimulating the repair of damaged DNA and triggering apoptosis of severely compromised cells.

The retinoblastoma tumor suppressor (pRb) and related pocket proteins, p107 and p130, are important regulatory subunits of the E2F transcription family members, which control cellular differentiation and proliferation.[25] The ability of E6 and E7 to disrupt the functions of p53 and pRb, respectively, is thus necessary for promoting proliferation and uncoupling differentiation. These cellular interactions, in turn, are able to keep the differentiating keratinocytes in a DNA replicative state, which is essential for progression of the HPV life cycle. However, these same processes can lead to transformation of the cell when left unregulated, such as occurs after the physical integration of high-risk HPV viral genomes into a host chromosome.

In high-risk HPVs, the E6 protein complexes with the E3 ubiquitin ligase, E6AP, and targets the p53 protein for ubiquitin-mediated proteosomal degradation.[17] It is the level of p53 breakdown that correlates with transformation risk. Both high-risk and low-risk E6 are able to bind p53, although only high-risk E6 proteins promote its degradation.[26] This functional difference between high-risk and low-risk E6 is explained by the binding of these proteins to different regions within p53.[27] Both high-risk and low-risk E6 proteins interact with the C-terminal domain of p53, but only high-risk E6 contacts the p53 core domain, an interaction that likely mediates the degradation of p53.[28] The high-risk E7 protein binds the retinoblastoma family of proteins (pRb, p107, and p130) and also induces their proteolytic degradation, which in turn allows for cell immortalization and helps to overcome DNA damage arrest signals.[29] Thus, cells expressing E7 are able to enter S phase in the absence of growth factors and despite the presence of inhibitory signals. High-risk E7 proteins have a greater transformation potential than low-risk E7 proteins, which correlates with the higher binding affinity of the high-risk E7 proteins for pRb.[25,30]

HPV histology
Histologically, HPV appears as a pedunculated mass with fingerlike projections or multiple fronds with a central fibrovascular core covered by stratified squamous epithelium.[31] The laryngeal mucosa appears velvety when papillomas remain microscopic, which is in contrast with the typical pinkish-whitish cauliflower presentation seen in the exophytic form. HPV also leads to a delay in epithelial maturation resulting in basal layer thickening and increased presence of nucleated cells in the suprabasal layer of the stratified epithelium.[32]

Molecular Mechanisms of RRP Disease

Although there are limited studies dealing with the molecular pathophysiology of the HPV types involved in RRP, there is a wealth of epidemiologic and molecular data on high-risk HPV types implicated as causing cervical cancers and a subset of head and neck cancers.[33,34] Cervical carcinomas harbor integrated high-risk HPV genomes within each tumor cell and continue to express the E6 and E7 viral oncogenes. As previously discussed, the high-risk E6 and E7 proteins modify the expression patterns and activities of many cellular genes and proteins to promote cell proliferation. It has been shown that both the E6 and E7 high-risk proteins are necessary for efficient immortalization of human keratinocytes.[25]

At the molecular level, much is known about the E6 and E7 oncoproteins of the high-risk HPVs, as discussed previously. In addition to binding the retinoblastoma family of proteins (pRb, p107, and p130) and targeting them for degradation, high-risk E7 is able to bind histone deacetylase (HDAC). Together, these activities allow cell immortalization and help to overcome DNA damage arrest signals.[29,35,36] High-risk HPV E7-expressing cells have also been shown to stabilize and increase the half-life of p53,[37,38] either by disrupting the p53-specific ubiquitin ligase mdm2[39] or by E2F-mediated transcriptional induction of p14ARF.[40] Furthermore, high-risk E7 is able to abrogate the cytostatic activities of certain cytokines important for restricting cellular growth and mounting an immune response to viral infection, such as transforming growth factor β (TGF-β), tumor necrosis factor α (TNF-α), IFN-α and IFN-γ, and insulin-like growth factors (IGFs). TGF-β, which is important for restricting epithelial cell growth, is resisted by high-risk E7 expression[41] and occurs in parallel with the acquisition of resistance to differentiation cues in E7-expressing keratinocytes.[42] TNF-β, an important mediator of immune response produced by cytotoxic T cells, also induces G1 growth arrest and cellular differentiation in normal keratinocytes. HPV E7-expressing keratinocytes continue to proliferate in the presence of TNF-β.[43] IFNs are produced in response to viral infections. HPV E7 can subvert the cellular response to IFNs by disrupting either IFN-α–mediated cellular signaling[44] or by downregulating the expression of IFN-β.[45–47] In addition, E7 can interact with insulinlike growth factor–binding protein-3,[48] and thus control the cellular availability of IGFs.

In addition to targeting p53 for degradation, high-risk E6 possesses redundant mechanisms for inactivating p53 and apoptosis. High-risk E6 can bind to p300, which blocks p53 acetylation and inhibits its ability to transactivate gene expression.[49] Also, E6 proteins target the proapoptotic effector, Bak, for proteolytic degradation,[50,51] thus inhibiting the intrinsic apoptosis pathway. High-risk E6 is also capable of inhibiting the extrinsic apoptosis pathway stimulated by both the Fas and the TNF-related apoptosis-inducing ligand (TRAIL) pathways. This inhibition is mediated by E6 binding to, and degradation of, both the Fas-associated protein with death domain (FADD) adapter protein and the effector caspase, caspase-8.[52] Furthermore, it has been observed that cells expressing the high-risk E6 proteins display a reduced ability to repair DNA damage.[53,54] Because the repair of DNA damage depends, at least in part, on the p53 status of cell, this may be caused by these E6-expressing cells being functionally p53 null.[55] Despite the inability to degrade p53, the E6 protein from a range of cutaneous HPV types effectively inhibits apoptosis in response to genotoxic ultraviolet (UV) damage.[56] This may partially be explained by the ability of E6 proteins to attenuate the UV-induced transactivation of p53-regulated proapoptotic genes *Fas*, *PUMA*, *Apaf-1*, and *PIG3*.[57] Further evidence of the ability of high-risk E6 to abrogate p53 function is by activating the transcription of ΔNP73, an isoform of the p53-related protein p73, which in turn inhibits the capacity of p53 to induce the transcription of genes involved in growth suppression and apoptosis.[58] In addition, high-risk E6 is able to induce telomerase activity in keratinocytes, which does not rely on p53 interaction but does require E6AP and is important for extending the life span of infected cells and their subsequent immortalization.[59,60]

By comparison, low-risk E6 and E7 proteins are usually included in molecular studies of high-risk HPV types because of their general lack of such abilities. For example, the E6 and E7 proteins of low-risk HPVs do not seem to express cell-transforming activities that are comparable with those of their high-risk counterparts.[30,61] It is also well known that the ability to promote the degradation of p53 is restricted to high-risk HPV types.[62] In addition, low-risk E7 binds to pRb family members with lower affinity than high-risk E7[25] and does not target pRb for degradation.[63] Despite these differences in function, the low-risk E6 and E7 proteins share significant homology with the high-risk proteins[64,65] and retain many of the same abilities that provide redundant mechanisms for promoting cellular proliferation, disrupting apoptosis, and uncoupling cellular differentiation.

Conserved E6 functions

Both HPV-16 and HPV-11 E6 proteins bind TRIP-Br1 (transcriptional integrator of the E2F1/DP1/RB cell cycle regulatory pathway). TRIP-Br1 modulates transcription of genes relevant for G1/S transition in the same direction as the E7 protein, through disruption of E2F1 transcriptional regulation. This redundancy in function shows important similarities between high-risk and low-risk E6 proteins that are important for both the HPV life cycle and potential cellular transformation.[66] In addition, high-risk and low-risk E6 proteins from HPV-16, HPV-18, and HPV-11 destabilize TIP60 (Tat-interacting protein 60 kDa), which relieves cellular promoters from TIP60 repression and abrogates p53-dependent activation of the apoptotic pathway. Degradation of TIP60, therefore, allows low-risk and high-risk HPVs to promote cell proliferation and cell survival.[67] Furthermore, HPV-16 and HPV-11 E6 proteins also bind and inactivate p73, which, at the least, promotes cell growth and may contribute to cellular transformation.[68] In addition, the ability to degrade the proapoptotic Bcl-2 family member, Bak, is conserved in high-risk and low-risk E6-expressing cells.[55,69] This ability to circumvent apoptosis is important for the HPV life cycle and presumably its transformation potential.

Conserved E7 functions

HPV-6, HPV-16, and HPV-18 E7 proteins interact with PCAF (P300/calcium-binding protein–associated factor) acetyltransferase, which is a coactivator for a variety of transcription factors including p53,[70] and thereby contributes to altered cellular gene expression and growth. Also, the E7 proteins from both high-risk and low-risk HPV types 16 and 11 interact with p300 and abolish p300-mediated E2 transactivation, which is important for differentiation-dependent activation of viral gene expression and potential cellular transformation.[71] In addition, both high-risk and low-risk E7 proteins (16, 18, 31, and 11) bind hypoxia-inducible factor 1α (HIF-1α) and enhance HIF-1α activity via displacement of HDACs. This mechanism is important for promoting epithelial growth through activation of angiogenesis. Furthermore, introduction of either high-risk or low-risk E7 genes (18 and 6) into epithelial raft cultures induces proliferating cell nuclear antigen (PCNA) expression in suprabasal cells, which indicates the importance of the E7 protein in reactivating host DNA replication machinery in differentiated, noncycling cells.[72] In addition, HPV-6 E7, like HPV-16 E7, interacts with and decreases the levels of p130, despite being unable to degrade other retinoblastoma tumor suppressor protein family members (pRb and p107). The ability of E7 proteins to destabilize the pRb family members depends on cellular differentiation, because both high-risk and low-risk E7 destabilize p130 in either differentiated or undifferentiated growth conditions. Only high-risk 16E7 degrades pRb in both growth conditions, whereas p107 is only destabilized by 16E7 in undifferentiated conditions.[73] The degradation of p130 is therefore likely necessary to complete the virus life cycle, whereas the added ability of 16E7 to regulate pRb and p107 may be related to oncogenic activity.

Immune responses

Another area of molecular interest is the complex innate and adaptive immune responses made by the host with respect to HPV-6 and HPV-11 infection. It remains unclear why only a small fraction of HPV-exposed individuals develop RRP, and why still fewer develop a severe course of the disease. One explanation proposes that patients with RRP are unable to produce an effective HPV-specific T-cell response, as shown by an altered $CD8^+$ subset and the T_H1/T_H2 cytokine imbalance found in these patients.[74] Supportive evidence for this theory later came from comparing relative gene expression levels between papilloma and adjacent normal tissue with respect to immune responsive genes using microarray analysis.[75] Additional studies revealed that HPV-11 E6 skews IL-10 and IFN-γ expression by patients with RRP toward increased IL-10 expression (T_H2) and away from IFN-γ (T_H1), which may be explained by an E6-induced dendritic cell dysfunction in these patients that shifts their HPV-specific immune responses toward IL-10 expression.[76] Further evidence of a dysfunctional immune response by patients with RRP is the finding that the transporter associated with antigen presentation (TAP-1) is downregulated along with the major histocompatibility complex (MHC) class I antigen in benign papillomas. TAP-1 protein expression correlated inversely with the frequency of disease recurrence. These findings suggest that HPV may evade immune recognition by decreasing the MHC cell surface expression via downregulation of TAP-1.[77]

Transmission of HPV

HPV is considered to be the most common sexually transmitted infection in the United States.[78] HPV prevalence has been gradually increasing in the female population. It is estimated that the overall prevalence of HPV in women aged 14 to 59 years is 26.8%. When analyzing smaller age groups, there is a prevalence of nearly 45% in women between the ages of 20 and 24 years.[79] These numbers also increase when factors such as education, poverty index, and marital status are taken into consideration. The prevalence increases in lower socioeconomic individuals, especially when they are unmarried and have not completed high school.[79] In addition, one study showed that the prevalence of HPV-6 or HPV-11 in sexually active women from 18 to 25 years of age was 2.2%, whereas the prevalence of HPV-16 or HPV-18 in the same cohort was 7.8%.[80]

Mother-to-child HPV transmission

Being a sexually transmitted disease, it has been hypothesized that HPV is transmitted vertically from the mother to the neonate during passage through the birth canal. However, this method has not been shown conclusively as the only mechanism for HPV infection. It has been shown that children born to mothers with active condylomata have an increased risk of infection, as much as 231 times that of disease-free mothers.[81] Additional risk of infection occurs when affected primigravid mothers have prolonged vaginal deliveries, especially with an increased duration after rupture of the membrane. Such an occurrence is thought to cause further risk because the neonate spends a greater amount of time exposed to the virus. The same study showed that the risk increased to nearly double if labor lasted for greater than 10 hours. It has also been suggested that newly acquired HPV infections tend to have greater infectivity compared with chronic infections.[82] These 2 factors alone show why low socioeconomic status (a group that has an increased prevalence of HPV) and age of the mother (increased likelihood of new-onset HPV and prolonged labor) are key risk factors for a neonate to develop RRP.

Although this knowledge helps to show the correlation between children with RRP and mothers with HPV, it implies a higher prevalence of this disease in children. However, despite how common HPV infections and active condylomata are in child-bearing women, RRP is an uncommon disease entity. Further, the odds of a child contracting HPV from a mother with active condylomata have been estimated at around 1 in 400,[83] which again suggests additional risk factors. Therefore, other factors seem likely to be important in the development of RRP: patient immunity; timing, length, and volume of virus exposure; and local traumas (intubation, extra-esophageal reflux).[7] In addition, neonates may become infected before birth, as evidenced by a recent study showing that approximately 12% of neonates may develop HPV infections through transplacental transmission.[84]

Caesarean section for HPV transmittal prevention

The hypothesis that HPV is transmitted to the neonate during transit through the birth canal has raised the question of whether caesarean section (C-section) may provide some degree of protection against transmission of HPV. A recent systematic review of literature was undertaken to answer this question.[85] The investigators showed that there was no statistically significant difference between the rates of HPV transmission from HPV-positive mothers either through vaginal delivery or C-section. Of the 6 selected studies, 3[86–88] showed no difference, whereas 3 studies[89–91] did show a decrease in HPV transmission with C-section. Tseng and colleagues[90] only included women with an intact amniotic sac before undergoing surgery in the C-section group. All women with rupture of membranes before C-section were excluded because these neonates may have been exposed to the virus in the window period between rupture of the amniotic sac and time of C-section. With these criteria for the C-section group, their results still showed a significant increase in HPV transmission with vaginal delivery compared with C-section, with a number needed to treat of only 5. The findings in this study correlate with other data[91] showing that membrane rupture even 2 hours before delivery (vaginal or C-section) increases the risk of HPV transmission.

Because prolonged exposure to HPV following rupture of the membrane can be bypassed through a C-section, it is possible that the difference between transmission rates among each type of delivery may increase when this aspect is considered. Although a planned C-section is a routine procedure, it still carries inherent surgical risks and results in increased morbidity and mortality for the mother.[7] Further studies are needed to determine the benefit of a planned C-section in an HPV-positive pregnant woman; however, it is a topic worthy of discussion between an at-risk mother and her birth care provider.

HPV vaccine

The recent advent of the HPV vaccine is encouraging, in that it will undoubtedly affect the spread of this disease. There are currently 2 vaccines present on the market. Cervarix, a European-approved product of Glaxo-Smith-Kline, is a bivalent vaccine designed against the L1 capsid proteins of HPV-16 and HPV-18, the 2 most common causes of cervical cancer. However, although vaccination against HPV-16 and HPV-18 may help prevent cervical cancer, this vaccine does not address HPV-6 and HPV-11, the most common causes of RRP. Gardasil is a prophylactic quadrivalent vaccine with activity against HPV-6, HPV-11, HPV-16, and HPV-18. It includes recombinant virus–like particles designed from the L1 capsid protein of the 4 different HPV types. A product of Merck, it was implemented on June 8, 2006, by the US Food and Drug Administration following the findings in the phase III study and several phase II studies that prompted the Advisory Committee on Immunization Practices (ACIP) to recommend its use.[92] Further, it was recommended that all girls 11 to 12 years old, and even as young as 9 years old, be given the vaccine along with women aged 13 to 26 years.[93]

Although there has been a growing negative response from parents toward vaccination because of the social stigma of the disease, HPV vaccination provides an overwhelming benefit for high-risk individuals. More importantly, preventative vaccination must be administered before sexual debut regardless of age, which further raises parental concerns. About 13% of American girls are sexually experienced by 15 years, and this number increases to 43% by age 17 years and 70% by age 19 years.[94] Also, the increase of teenage pregnancy compounds the problem of potential neonatal transmission of HPV. So although the concept of preventative vaccination of HPV seems straightforward from a medical perspective, the underlying social issues are problematic.

In addition, the vaccine has also been approved for treatment in men. The idea of vaccinating boys has been embraced by other countries, such as Australia, where it is available to boys from the age of 9 to 15 years.[95] HPV infection among men seems to be as common as in women but is often asymptomatic, which contributes to the high rate of transmission between sexual partners.[96] Because of its silent presentation, HPV transmission during heterosexual contact can occur without either partner being aware. The proponents of administering the vaccine to boys hope that the vaccination of both girls and boys will help slow the spread of the major serotypes of HPV.

Although each individual benefits from vaccination, it is uncertain what effect this will have on neonatal transmission of HPV or on the overall incidence of RRP. For an individual neonate, there may be an added benefit from vaccination in conjunction with performing C-section before rupture of the amniotic sac. It has been suggested that vaccines might eventually be useful in neonates for 2 reasons: (1) via transmission of immunity through maternal antibodies, and (2) through direct vaccination of neonates similar to hepatitis B neonatal vaccination.[97] Currently, HPV vaccines are not approved for routine use on neonates, so this application requires further research.

The concept of herd immunity through vaccination of at-risk individuals should also be considered. The basis of this belief is that all women, and likely all men, from a specific age group within the population will be vaccinated. The number of those vaccinated eventually overwhelms those who are infected. As subsequent generations continue to be vaccinated, those vaccinated individuals will theoretically provide the community with immunity against the disease. Ideally, once such a community status exists, there will also be a consequent decrease in incidence of disease, in this case RRP. With these theories in mind, the HPV vaccine promises to decrease the future incidence of RRP; however, this needs further testing.

Clinical Manifestations of RRP

General respiratory symptoms in RRP
Despite becoming infected either before or during birth, most pediatric patients do not manifest any symptoms of RRP immediately. The larynx is the most common site of

infection in children and, therefore, presenting symptoms tend to reflect this fact. As expected with laryngeal involvement, hoarseness is the first symptom noted; however, because of the subtle nature of this finding in a child, much less an infant, clinical suspicion for a disease process rarely arises.[98] Other symptoms, secondary to upper airway involvement, may include dyspnea, chronic cough, recurrent upper respiratory infections, pneumonia, acute respiratory distress, dysphagia, and/or failure to thrive.[2] Stridor, initially inspiratory and then biphasic, can be the presenting symptom of RRP and warrants significant clinical suspicion for disease and the appropriate work-up, including examination of the larynx and upper airway.

Delay in diagnosing RRP

Without a reason to suspect RRP, many patients are initially assumed to have a more common respiratory problem, such as croup, asthma, or bronchitis. Depending on the age of the child and based on the symptoms discussed earlier, allergies, acid reflux, and/or vocal fold nodules are often included in the differential diagnosis and worked up appropriately. Because of a low index of suspicion and subtle presenting signs, the definitive diagnosis of RRP is often made around 1 year after initial symptoms began.[3,99] RRP is most commonly diagnosed between 2 and 4 years of age, with dysphonia being the most common presenting complaint.[100,101] Most juvenile patients with RRP (75%) are diagnosed by age 5 years.[7]

Variable course of RRP

As a highly unpredictable disease, RRP can vary in course with each affected patient. In a percentage of patients, the disease is aggressive and requires frequent debridement to protect from airway compromise. In contrast, select patients may show a progressive and sometimes spontaneous remission. Although these 2 extremes are noted, most tend to exhibit a course that lies somewhere in the middle. The course of RRP in certain patients may be further affected by the introduction of a tracheotomy or endotracheal tube. Despite the benefits of providing a secure airway, irritation and disruption of normal mucosa by these tubes increases the risk of spreading papillomas into the subglottis and proximal trachea. Nearly 30% of affected children manifest extralaryngeal spread of RRP.[102] The most common site is the oral cavity followed by trachea, bronchi, and then esophagus.[3,98,102] In some rare cases, the larynx may be completely unaffected, despite the presence of tracheal disease.[103]

Pulmonary spread of RRP can be identified on computed tomography (CT) as noncalcified peripheral nodules that show central cavitation and air-fluid levels. Patients with pulmonary RRP incur perhaps the most aggressive course of the disease. Beginning initially with recurrent pneumonias and bronchiectasis, these patients eventually progress to frank pulmonary failure caused by destruction of underlying lung parenchyma as the disease progresses. In severe cases, malignant transformation of RRP into SCCA occurs.[102] This typically fatal presentation is rare, accounting for less than 1% of disease presentations and is usually associated with HPV-11 infection.[104,105] **Figs. 1–4** show varying presentations of RRP.

> **PEARLS & PITFALLS:** *Because of the risk of malignant conversion, it is necessary to take adequate biopsies periodically during subsequent procedures and monitor for any concerning pulmonary changes.*

Staging of RRP is integral for both the clinician's knowledge of the progress of the disease as well as for clear communication of the patient's status to another physician. Although various staging schemes exist, they share certain principles. One of the more commonly used staging systems assigns numeric scores for a combination of

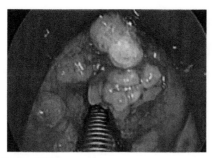

Fig. 1. Various presentations of RRP.

subjective and objective findings.[106,107] In the subjective portion, the patient's level of respiratory distress, stridor, urgency of intervention, and voice are qualified. In addition, an aspect of a surgical timeframe may be included by charting the time between surgeries and number of surgeries in a specific time period. The second half of the assessment is a quantification of the disease through the use of laryngoscopy. It entails assessing the extent of the lesion (small surface lesion to large bulky lesion) and the locations of the lesions. Typically, the locations are separated according to subsites within the larynx, subsites in the trachea, and an extra category for presence of lesions elsewhere. The most important aspect of staging is including an extensive level of detail when recording the objective laryngoscopic findings. Once staged, the need for treatment can be assessed and the evaluation of the prior intervention can be determined. This information is particularly useful when adjuvant therapy is being used, and benefits of the medications need to be balanced against potential toxicities (**Fig. 5**).

> *Pearls & Pitfalls: Implementation of a staging system allows for the practitioner to make an accurate comparison of the patient's disease between visits and to clearly communicate the disease severity with other physicians.*

Treatment of Recurrent Respiratory Papilloma

The treatment of RRP largely consists of surgical management, often augmented by the use of pharmacotherapy. Surgical treatment consists of debulking the papillomas to secure a stable airway while preserving the underlying laryngeal tissues. Surgery is often performed via microscopic or endoscopic rigid laryngoscopy in the operating room using either a laser or microdebrider to remove papillomas. A variety of lasers

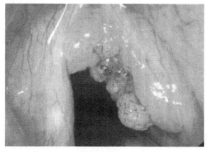

Fig. 2. Various presentations of RRP.

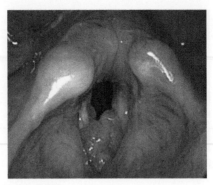

Fig. 3. Various presentations of RRP.

have been used for this purpose, including CO2, KTP (potassium titanyl phosphate), and pulse-dyed lasers. Although lasers remain the traditional standard, the use of microdebriders has been gaining favor. The reason for this trend is the ability of the microdebrider to selectively suction the affected tissue, which often allows for more precise debridement, limited damage to the underlying tissues, and greater preservation of normal epithelium. These characteristics become increasingly important because of the nature of RRP, which often necessitates several visits to the operating room for debulking, with an average of 4.1 to 4.4 surgeries during the first year of diagnosis alone.[6] See **Figs. 6** and **7** for preoperative and postoperative surgical intervention for laryngeal lesions and see Video 1 on the technique of microdebrider for removal of papillomas.

>*Pearls & Pitfalls: With the specially designed blade for the microdebrider, lesions can be separated through use of suction from benign laryngeal tissue during resection, without need for cold dissection.*

Surgical treatment of RRP

Among surgical options, a tracheotomy may be performed, but it is typically reserved for those most aggressive cases with impending airway compromise. Although this procedure may be necessary to secure an airway, it does provide another site for rapid colonization and serves as a conduit for disease spread to the tracheobronchial tree.[1] In a series studying patients with RRP in whom a tracheotomy was performed, tracheal papillomas were present in more than half of those patients.[108] Therefore, it

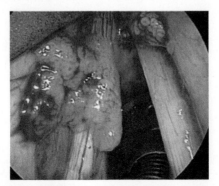

Fig. 4. Various presentations of RRP.

STAGING ASSESSMENT FOR RECURRENT LARYNGEAL PAPILOMATOSIS

PATIENT INNITIALS: ___ DATE OF SURGERY: ___ SURGEON: ____
PATIENT ID#: ___   INSTITUTION:____

1. How long since the last papilloma surgery? ___days, ___weeks, ___months, ___years,

   ___don't know, ___1st surgery

2. Counting today's surgery, how many papilloma surgeries in the past 12 months? ___

3. Describe the patient's voice today: ____normal (0), ___ abnormal (1), ___aphonic (2)

4. Describe the patient's stridor today: ___absent (0), ___present with activity (1), ___present at rest (2)

5. Describe the urgency of today's intervention: ___scheduled (0), ___elective (1), ___urgent (2),
   ___emergent (3)

6. Describe today's level of respiratory distress: ___ none (0), ___ mild (1), ___ moderate (2),
   ___ severe (3), ___ extreme (4)

TOTAL SCORE for questions 3-6: ___

FOR EACH SITE, SCORE AS: 0 = none, 1 = surface lesion, 2 = raised lesion, 3 = bulky lesion

LARYNX

   Epiglottis
       Lingual surface _____**Laryngeal surface** _____
       Aryepiglottic folds: Right____   **Left**____
       False vocal cords: Right____   **Left**____
       True vocal cords: Right____   **Left**____
       Arytenoids: Right____   **Left**____
       Subglottis ___   **Posterior commissure** ___
                                  Anterior commissure ___

TRACHEA:
       Upper one-third ___
       Middle one-third ___
       Lower one-third ___
       Bronchi: Right ___ **Left** ___
       Trachcotomy stoma___

OTHER
       Nose ___
       Palate ___
       Pharynx ___
       Lungs ___
       Other ___

TOTAL SCORE ALL SITES: _____

Fig. 5. Coltrera-Derkay staging and severity scheme. (*From* Derkay CS, Malis DJ, Zalzal G, et al. A staging system for assessing severity of disease and response to therapy in recurrent respiratory papillomatosis. Laryngoscope 1998;108:936; with permission.)

is widely accepted now that tracheotomy should be reserved for only those cases in which multiple debulking surgeries have failed and/or the child's airway becomes compromised. Furthermore, if a tracheotomy is unavoidable, decannulation should be considered as early as possible once the disease process is controlled and the airway is deemed stable.

Adjuvant therapy for RRP

Adjuvant pharmacotherapy for the treatment of RRP continues to be an area of exploratory interest, with several agents currently used that work by varying mechanisms.

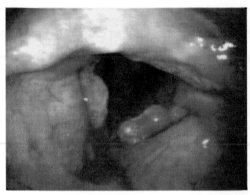

Fig. 6. Pre-treatment initial presentation of laryngeal papillomas in a 37 year-old female patient.

One example is (IFN-α, a human leukocyte protein produced by the body naturally in response to viral infections. Although its exact mechanism of action in RRP is not well understood, its natural role in the immune response is to bind cell receptors and modulate the cell's metabolism, leading to antiproliferative and immune-protective effects. The benefits of this therapy must also be weighed against the toxicities of IFN-α, which include thrombocytopenia and leukopenia. In addition, systemic symptoms, such as fevers, fatigue, nausea, arthralgia, and headache, make prolonged therapy difficult for the patient.

A recent multicenter study comparing surgery alone versus surgery with adjuvant IFN-α showed an initial decrease in disease progression at 6 months.[109] However, this effect did not persist after 2 years, and no benefit was observed from the use of adjuvant IFN-α rather than surgery alone. A different study showed that continuous use of IFN-α resulted in a response rate of 75% with a third of patients undergoing complete remission of their disease. The proposed algorithm by Leventhal and colleagues[110] is to start with the use of IFN-α for 6 months then reevaluate the disease response. Prolonged use is encouraged if a positive response is noted; however, treatment should be halted if no response is noted or toxicities develop. An increased

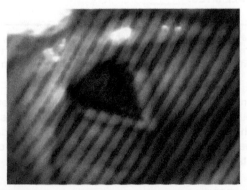

Fig. 7. 3 month post-treatment photo of 37 year old patient with new onset laryngeal papillomas (seen in **Fig. 6**). Treatment included microsurgical debridement of papillomas and aggressive anti-reflux therapy with twice daily proton pump inhibitors.

response to IFN-α in patients with HPV-6 compared with HPV-11 disease may also exist.[111] Although its exact benefit is unpredictable, IFN-α remains a cornerstone in adjuvant therapy for RRP.

Among antiviral agents, cidofovir is the most used agent. Ribavirin has been used sparsely and has not shown any clear aid in disease suppression.[112] Cidofovir, as an analogue of cytosine, has antiviral activity against DNA viruses. Its effects are induction of apoptosis and augmentation of the immune system, although the exact mechanism is not well understood.[113] Cidofovir may be used either through traditional intralesional injections or, more recently, inhalation.[114] Intralesional injections of cidofovir at the time of surgery have been tested in prospective studies that showed partial to complete regression of papillomas and a decrease in the frequency of debulking surgeries.[115–121] A benefit of intralesional injections is that a higher concentration can be reached locally without greatly increasing plasma levels.[121] Despite this advantage, the toxicities of intravenous use of cidofovir in humans should be considered, and include nephrotoxicity, bone marrow toxicity, iritis, and uveitis.[122] Its off label use should be cautioned against because cidofovir has been found to be carcinogenic, embryotoxic, and teratogenic in animals.[123] Despite these harmful effects, a review of literature discussing cidofovir as adjuvant therapy showed that greater 80% of patients show either partial or complete response.[124] The caveat to these positive findings is that no statistically significant study has yet been performed comparing surgical debridement plus cidofovir with surgical debridement plus placebo.

Other recent agents include indole-3-carbinol (I3C), HSP E7, mumps vaccine, and photodynamic therapy (PDT). I3C is derived from cruciferous vegetables and has shown promise in vitro by decreasing papilloma growth through manipulation of estrogen metabolism. In a small clinical trial of 9 patients, 4 patients had partial or complete response with no negative effects.[125] HSP E7 is a recombinant protein combining heat shock protein 65 of *Mycobacterium bovis* and the E7 protein of HPV-16. In a study of HSP E7 administered subcutaneously, a decrease in frequency of surgery and a decrease in the absolute number of surgical procedures were noted with mild reactions at the site of injection.[126]

Intralesional injections of the mumps vaccine has been tested and showed an increased length of remission in children, with low, if any, adverse effects.[127] In this case series, the author outlined the use of mumps vaccine injected at the base of a lesion before use of a CO_2 laser to remove the papillomas. Following a remission rate of greater than 80% in a small test group, a second, larger group was treated in a similar fashion with nearly identical results after a minimum of 2 years' follow-up. Despite this success, the study required a control group and a fixed algorithm to provide internal validity. The mumps vaccine has been used in cutaneous lesions to help generate a local inflammatory response, but this same principle has not been shown with RRP. Although this series reflects a pattern, the assumption of causality should not be made without a control. The use of intralesional mumps vaccine as an adjuvant therapy is an intriguing hypothesis, but it can only remain as such without a prospective, randomized trial to lend credence.[128]

PEARLS & PITFALLS: Although CO_2 laser was initially favored, its longer wavelength causes greater thermal injury to underlying tissue. The newer angiolytic KTP and pulse-dyed lasers cause less thermal damage without disruption of the basement membrane.

PDT for RRP

Photodynamic therapy (PDT) in the treatment of RRP has shown promise. The benefit of this modality to selectively treat tumor cells without causing damage to healthy

---

Note to the pediatrician: diagnosis of RRP

Because of the location of RRP, definitive diagnosis requires direct visualization of the upper airway. Although this ultimately requires otolaryngology referral, the primary care provider can play a significant role in early diagnosis. As discussed earlier, RRP can present with a multitude of symptoms, including hoarseness, chronic cough, dyspnea, recurrent upper respiratory infections, pneumonias, dysphagia, stridor, or failure to thrive. Because of the often subtle nature of initial symptoms, many diseases, some of which may be more acute or emergent, are often considered first. When a patient does not show timely improvement with appropriate therapy for these initial diagnoses, RRP should be considered as an alternate diagnosis. In this capacity, the primary care provider plays an essential role in the process by having a high index of suspicion, which leads to an earlier diagnosis and implementation of a treatment plan.

---

tissue makes this treatment unique.[129,130] PDT has been approved for use in lung cancer, esophageal cancer, and Barrett esophagus. RRP shares a similarity with these disorders in that the area of disease is superficial and has high cell turnover. PDT is used in conjunction with an injectable photosensitizer, such as Photofrin (Pc 4), which promotes apoptosis in cells after laser excitation. In the case of RRP, the PDT may provide benefit by altering the immune response, making it more sensitive to even low concentrations of viral proteins.[131,132] Currently, there are some discrepancies concerning the benefit of PDT, with some studies showing decreased papilloma growth and potential long-term effects, whereas others show limited benefits.[133–135] PDT remains an area of future study to better understand its mechanism of action as well as to evaluate its benefit as adjuvant therapy.

Laryngopharyngeal reflux treatment related to RRP

One additional area to mention in the treatment of RRP is the management of laryngopharyngeal reflux disease (LPRD). Irritation of the epithelium of the aerodigestive tract triggered by LPRD, either through acid or gastric enzyme interaction, may produce mucosal damage or an inflammatory response that could potentially trigger proliferation or spread of papilloma disease. Effective management of LPRD may result in improved control of RRP and possibly complete remission.[135–137] In a small group of pediatric patients, administration of antireflux therapy placed all patients into remission; however, a break in therapy resulted in the return of papillomas, requiring debridement.[137] Holland and colleagues[138] showed a decrease in frequency of patients with RRP forming laryngeal webs when treated with antireflux medications. Unlike some of the previously mentioned adjuvant therapies, antireflux medications carry fewer adverse side effects and also provide added benefits to patients with vocal dysfunction from RRP disease. Further trials are needed to objectively evaluate and quantify the role of antireflux therapy in RRP, but the initial studies exploring concurrent treatment of LPRD seem to show an added benefit.

SUMMARY ON RRP

RRP is a benign disease of the upper aerodigestive tract caused by infection with HPV, and can have potentially life-threatening airway compromise and a protracted clinical course. The clinical course of this disease entity can be challenging for several reasons. In pediatric populations, the presenting symptoms are often nonspecific and subtle, which frequently results in a delayed diagnosis. Generally, the disease process is unpredictable, ranging from mild disease and spontaneous remission to an aggressive disease with pulmonary spread and requirements for frequent debulking procedures. In severe cases, the uncontrolled proliferation of papillomas can result in airway compromise and the need for an emergent airway. However, the procedure to establish an airway may lead to distal spread of the disease and additional surgeries. Because there is no known cure, multiple surgical debridements have become the mainstay of treatment. Advanced instrumentation, such as the microdebrider and newer angiolytic lasers (KTP, pulse-dyed laser), has allowed more precise removal and thus easier preservation of delicate laryngeal tissues, with improved voice results. Although considered rare, this disease entity is potentially devastating and costly to patients, families, and society in general, which highlights its clinical relevance.

Although studies of the molecular mechanisms and pathophysiology of low-risk HPVs are limited, this is an area primed for innovation. Major strides have been achieved in this field already with the development of the HPV vaccine, which shows promise for reducing the prevalence of RRP, in addition to eliminating cervical cancer. Advancing the basic science and clinical translational research made available from studying the high-risk HPV types carries the potential for new discoveries and novel therapies for RRP.

REFERENCES

1. Tasca RA, Clarke RW. Recurrent respiratory papillomatosis. Arch Dis Child 2006;91(8):689–91.
2. Derkay CS, Wiatrak B. Recurrent respiratory papillomatosis: a review. Laryngoscope 2008;118(7):1236–47.
3. Derkay CS. Task force on recurrent respiratory papillomas. A preliminary report. Arch Otolaryngol Head Neck Surg 1995;121(12):1386–91.
4. Marsico M, Mehta V, Wentworth C, et al. Estimating the disease burden of juvenile onset RRP in the US using large administrative databases – preliminary pilot results [abstract P-03.58]. Presented May 2009 at the International Papillomavirus Conference. Available at: http://www.hpv2009.org. Accessed May, 2009.
5. Leung R, Hawkes M, Campisi P. Severity of juvenile onset recurrent respiratory papillomatosis is not associated with socioeconomic status in a setting of universal health care. Int J Pediatr Otorhinolaryngol 2007;71(6):965–72.
6. Armstrong LR, Derkay CS, Reeves WC. Initial results from the national registry for juvenile-onset recurrent respiratory papillomatosis. RRP Task Force. Arch Otolaryngol Head Neck Surg 1999;125(7):743–8.
7. Larson DA, Derkay CS. Epidemiology of recurrent respiratory papillomatosis. APMIS 2010;118(6–7):450–4.
8. Ullman EV. On the aetiology of laryngeal papilloma. Acta Otolaryngol 1923;5:317.
9. Gissmann L, Wolnik L, Ikenberg H, et al. Human papillomavirus types 6 and 11 DNA sequences in genital and laryngeal papillomas and in some cervical cancers. Proc Natl Acad Sci U S A 1983;80(2):560–3.
10. Mounts P, Shah KV, Kashima H. Viral etiology of juvenile- and adult-onset squamous papilloma of the larynx. Proc Natl Acad Sci U S A 1982;79(17):5425–9 PMCID: PMC346910.
11. Gabbott M, Cossart YE, Kan A, et al. Human papillomavirus and host variables as predictors of clinical course in patients with juvenile-onset recurrent respiratory papillomatosis. J Clin Microbiol 1997;35(12):3098–103.
12. Pou AM, Rimell FL, Jordan JA, et al. Adult respiratory papillomatosis: human papillomavirus type and viral coinfections as predictors of prognosis. Ann Otol Rhinol Laryngol 1995;104(10 Pt 1):758–62.
13. Duggan MA, Lim M, Gill MJ, et al. HPV DNA typing of adult-onset respiratory papillomatosis. Laryngoscope 1990;100(6):639–42.

14. Major T, Szarka K, Sziklai I, et al. The characteristics of human papillomavirus DNA in head and neck cancers and papillomas. J Clin Pathol 2005;58(1): 51–5. PMCID: PMC1770542.
15. Derkay CS, Darrow DH. Recurrent respiratory papillomatosis. Ann Otol Rhinol Laryngol 2006;115(1):1–11.
16. Hartley C, Hamilton J, Birzgalis AR, et al. Recurrent respiratory papillomatosis– the Manchester experience, 1974-1992. J Laryngol Otol 1994;108(3):226–9.
17. Donne AJ, Hampson L, Homer JJ, et al. The role of HPV type in recurrent respiratory papillomatosis. Int J Pediatr Otorhinolaryngol 2010;74(1):7–14.
18. Gorgoulis V, Rassidakis G, Karameris A, et al. Expression of p53 protein in laryngeal squamous cell carcinoma and dysplasia: possible correlation with human papillomavirus infection and clinicopathological findings. Virchows Arch 1994; 425(5):481–9.
19. Majoros M, Devine KD, Parkhill EM. Malignant transformation of benign laryngeal papillomas in children after radiation therapy. Surg Clin North Am 1963; 43:1049–61.
20. Reidy PM, Dedo HH, Rabah R, et al. Integration of human papillomavirus type 11 in recurrent respiratory papilloma-associated cancer. Laryngoscope 2004; 114(11):1906–9.
21. Go C, Schwartz MR, Donovan DT. Molecular transformation of recurrent respiratory papillomatosis: viral typing and p53 overexpression. Ann Otol Rhinol Laryngol 2003;112(4):298–302.
22. Miller CS, Johnstone BM. Human papillomavirus as a risk factor for oral squamous cell carcinoma: a meta-analysis, 1982-1997. Oral Surg Oral Med Oral Pathol Oral Radiol Endod 2001;91(6):622–35.
23. Smith EM, Pignatari SS, Gray SD, et al. Human papillomavirus infection in papillomas and nondiseased respiratory sites of patients with recurrent respiratory papillomatosis using the polymerase chain reaction. Arch Otolaryngol Head Neck Surg 1993;119(5):554–7.
24. Stern Y, Felipovich A, Cotton RT, et al. Immunocompetency in children with recurrent respiratory papillomatosis: prospective study. Ann Otol Rhinol Laryngol 2007;116(3):169–71.
25. Munger K, Phelps WC, Bubb V, et al. The E6 and E7 genes of the human papillomavirus type 16 together are necessary and sufficient for transformation of primary human keratinocytes. J Virol 1989;63(10):4417–21.
26. Scheffner M, Werness BA, Huibregtse JM, et al. The E6 oncoprotein encoded by human papillomavirus types 16 and 18 promotes the degradation of p53. Cell 1990;63(6):1129–36.
27. Li X, Coffino P. High-risk human papillomavirus E6 protein has two distinct binding sites within p53, of which only one determines degradation. J Virol 1996;70(7):4509–16.
28. Pietsch EC, Murphy ME. Low risk HPV-E6 traps p53 in the cytoplasm and induces p53-dependent apoptosis. Cancer Biol Ther 2008;7(12):1916–8.
29. Helt AM, Galloway DA. Mechanisms by which DNA tumor virus oncoproteins target the Rb family of pocket proteins. Carcinogenesis 2003;24(2):159–69.
30. Barbosa MS, Vass WC, Lowy DR, et al. In vitro biological activities of the E6 and E7 genes vary among human papillomaviruses of different oncogenic potential. J Virol 1991;65(1):292–8.
31. Abramson AL, Steinberg BM, Winkler B. Laryngeal papillomatosis: clinical, histopathologic and molecular studies. Laryngoscope 1987;97(6): 678–85.

32. Steinberg BM, Meade R, Kalinowski S, et al. Abnormal differentiation of human papillomavirus-induced laryngeal papillomas. Arch Otolaryngol Head Neck Surg 1990;116(10):1167–71.

33. Cogliano V, Baan R, Straif K, et al. Carcinogenicity of human papillomaviruses. Lancet Oncol 2005;6(4):204.

34. zur Hausen H. Papillomaviruses in human cancers. Proc Assoc Am Physicians 1999;111(6):581–7.

35. Helt AM, Funk JO, Galloway DA. Inactivation of both the retinoblastoma tumor suppressor and p21 by the human papillomavirus type 16 E7 oncoprotein is necessary to inhibit cell cycle arrest in human epithelial cells. J Virol 2002; 76(20):10559–68.

36. Longworth MS, Wilson R, Laimins LA. HPV31 E7 facilitates replication by activating E2F2 transcription through its interaction with HDACs. EMBO J 2005; 24(10):1821–30.

37. Demers GW, Halbert CL, Galloway DA. Elevated wild-type p53 protein levels in human epithelial cell lines immortalized by the human papillomavirus type 16 E7 gene. Virology 1994;198(1):169–74.

38. Jones DL, Thompson DA, Munger K. Destabilization of the RB tumor suppressor protein and stabilization of p53 contribute to HPV type 16 E7-induced apoptosis. Virology 1997;239(1):97–107.

39. Seavey SE, Holubar M, Saucedo LJ, et al. The E7 oncoprotein of human papillomavirus type 16 stabilizes p53 through a mechanism independent of p19(ARF). J Virol 1999;73(9):7590–8.

40. Bates S, Phillips AC, Clark PA, et al. p14ARF links the tumour suppressors RB and p53. Nature 1998;395(6698):124–5.

41. Pietenpol JA, Stein RW, Moran E, et al. TGF-beta 1 inhibition of c-myc transcription and growth in keratinocytes is abrogated by viral transforming proteins with pRB binding domains. Cell 1990;61(5):777–85.

42. Borger DR, Mi Y, Geslani G, et al. Retinoic acid resistance at late stages of human papillomavirus type 16-mediated transformation of human keratinocytes arises despite intact retinoid signaling and is due to a loss of sensitivity to transforming growth factor-beta. Virology 2000;270(2):397–407.

43. Munger K, Basile JR, Duensing S, et al. Biological activities and molecular targets of the human papillomavirus E7 oncoprotein. Oncogene 2001;20(54): 7888–98.

44. Barnard P, McMillan NA. The human papillomavirus E7 oncoprotein abrogates signaling mediated by interferon-alpha. Virology 1999;259(2):305–13.

45. Park JS, Kim EJ, Kwon HJ, et al. Inactivation of interferon regulatory factor-1 tumor suppressor protein by HPV E7 oncoprotein. Implication for the E7-mediated immune evasion mechanism in cervical carcinogenesis. J Biol Chem 2000;275(10):6764–9.

46. Brehm A, Nielsen SJ, Miska EA, et al. The E7 oncoprotein associates with Mi2 and histone deacetylase activity to promote cell growth. EMBO J 1999;18(9): 2449–58.

47. Luscher-Firzlaff JM, Westendorf JM, Zwicker J, et al. Interaction of the fork head domain transcription factor MPP2 with the human papilloma virus 16 E7 protein: enhancement of transformation and transactivation. Oncogene 1999;18(41): 5620–30.

48. Mannhardt B, Weinzimer SA, Wagner M, et al. Human papillomavirus type 16 E7 oncoprotein binds and inactivates growth-inhibitory insulin-like growth factor binding protein 3. Mol Cell Biol 2000;20(17):6483–95.

49. Patel D, Huang SM, Baglia LA, et al. The E6 protein of human papillomavirus type 16 binds to and inhibits co-activation by CBP and p300. EMBO J 1999; 18(18):5061–72.

50. Jackson S, Harwood C, Thomas M, et al. Role of Bak in UV-induced apoptosis in skin cancer and abrogation by HPV E6 proteins. Genes Dev 2000;14(23): 3065–73.

51. Thomas M, Pim D, Banks L. The role of the E6-p53 interaction in the molecular pathogenesis of HPV. Oncogene 1999;18(53):7690–700.

52. Filippova M, Parkhurst L, Duerksen-Hughes PJ. The human papillomavirus 16 E6 protein binds to Fas-associated death domain and protects cells from Fas-triggered apoptosis. J Biol Chem 2004;279(24):25729–44.

53. Finzer P, Aguilar-Lemarroy A, Rosl F. The role of human papillomavirus oncoproteins E6 and E7 in apoptosis. Cancer Lett 2002;188(1–2):15–24.

54. Giampieri S, Storey A. Repair of UV-induced thymine dimers is compromised in cells expressing the E6 protein from human papillomaviruses types 5 and 18. Br J Cancer 2004;90(11):2203–9.

55. Thomas M, Banks L. Human papillomavirus (HPV) E6 interactions with Bak are conserved amongst E6 proteins from high and low risk HPV types. J Gen Virol 1999;80(Pt 6):1513–7.

56. Jackson S, Storey A. E6 proteins from diverse cutaneous HPV types inhibit apoptosis in response to UV damage. Oncogene 2000;19(4):592–8.

57. Giampieri S, Garcia-Escudero R, Green J, et al. Human papillomavirus type 77 E6 protein selectively inhibits p53-dependent transcription of proapoptotic genes following UV-B irradiation. Oncogene 2004;23(34):5864–70.

58. Accardi R, Dong W, Smet A, et al. Skin human papillomavirus type 38 alters p53 functions by accumulation of deltaNp73. EMBO Rep 2006;7(3):334–40. PMCID: PMC1456898.

59. Klingelhutz AJ, Foster SA, McDougall JK. Telomerase activation by the E6 gene product of human papillomavirus type 16. Nature 1996;380(6569):79–82.

60. Gewin L, Myers H, Kiyono T, et al. Identification of a novel telomerase repressor that interacts with the human papillomavirus type-16 E6/E6-AP complex. Genes Dev 2004;18(18):2269–82.

61. Storey A, Osborn K, Crawford L. Co-transformation by human papillomavirus types 6 and 11. J Gen Virol 1990;71(Pt 1):165–71.

62. Storey A, Pim D, Murray A, et al. Comparison of the in vitro transforming activities of human papillomavirus types. EMBO J 1988;7(6):1815–20.

63. Demers GW, Foster SA, Halbert CL, et al. Growth arrest by induction of p53 in DNA damaged keratinocytes is bypassed by human papillomavirus 16 E7. Proc Natl Acad Sci U S A 1994;91(10):4382–6.

64. Nomine Y, Masson M, Charbonnier S, et al. Structural and functional analysis of E6 oncoprotein: insights in the molecular pathways of human papillomavirus-mediated pathogenesis. Mol Cell 2006;21(5):665–78.

65. Gage JR, Meyers C, Wettstein FO. The E7 proteins of the nononcogenic human papillomavirus type 6b (HPV-6b) and of the oncogenic HPV-16 differ in retinoblastoma protein binding and other properties. J Virol 1990;64(2):723–30.

66. Gupta S, Takhar PP, Degenkolbe R, et al. The human papillomavirus type 11 and 16 E6 proteins modulate the cell-cycle regulator and transcription cofactor TRIP-Br1. Virology 2003;317(1):155–64.

67. Jha S, Vande PS, Banerjee NS, et al. Destabilization of TIP60 by human papillomavirus E6 results in attenuation of TIP60-dependent transcriptional regulation and apoptotic pathway. Mol Cell 2010;38(5):700–11.

68. Park JS, Kim EJ, Lee JY, et al. Functional inactivation of p73, a homolog of p53 tumor suppressor protein, by human papillomavirus E6 proteins. Int J Cancer 2001;91(6):822–7.
69. Underbrink MP, Howie HL, Bedard KM, et al. E6 proteins from multiple human betapapillomavirus types degrade Bak and protect keratinocytes from apoptosis after UVB irradiation. J Virol 2008;82(21):10408–17.
70. Avvakumov N, Torchia J, Mymryk JS. Interaction of the HPV E7 proteins with the pCAF acetyltransferase. Oncogene 2003;22(25):3833–41.
71. Bernat A, Avvakumov N, Mymryk JS, et al. Interaction between the HPV E7 oncoprotein and the transcriptional coactivator p300. Oncogene 2003;22(39): 7871–81.
72. Cheng S, Schmidt-Grimminger DC, Murant T, et al. Differentiation-dependent up-regulation of the human papillomavirus E7 gene reactivates cellular DNA replication in suprabasal differentiated keratinocytes. Genes Dev 1995;9(19): 2335–49.
73. Zhang B, Chen W, Roman A. The E7 proteins of low- and high-risk human papillomaviruses share the ability to target the pRB family member p130 for degradation. Proc Natl Acad Sci U S A 2006;103(2):437–42.
74. Bonagura VR, Hatam L, DeVoti J, et al. Recurrent respiratory papillomatosis: altered CD8(+) T-cell subsets and T(H)1/T(H)2 cytokine imbalance. Clin Immunol 1999;93(3):302–11.
75. DeVoti JA, Rosenthal DW, Wu R, et al. Immune dysregulation and tumor-associated gene changes in recurrent respiratory papillomatosis: a paired microarray analysis. Mol Med 2008;14(9–10):608–17.
76. DeVoti JA, Steinberg BM, Rosenthal DW, et al. Failure of gamma interferon but not interleukin-10 expression in response to human papillomavirus type 11 E6 protein in respiratory papillomatosis. Clin Diagn Lab Immunol 2004;11(3):538–47.
77. Vambutas A, Bonagura VR, Steinberg BM. Altered expression of TAP-1 and major histocompatibility complex class I in laryngeal papillomatosis: correlation of TAP-1 with disease. Clin Diagn Lab Immunol 2000;7(1):79–85.
78. Weinstock H, Berman S, Cates W Jr. Sexually transmitted diseases among American youth: incidence and prevalence estimates, 2000. Perspect Sex Reprod Health 2004;36(1):6–10.
79. Dunne EF, Unger ER, Sternberg M, et al. Prevalence of HPV infection among females in the United States. JAMA 2007;297(8):813–9.
80. Manhart LE, Holmes KK, Koutsky LA, et al. Human papillomavirus infection among sexually active young women in the United States: implications for developing a vaccination strategy. Sex Transm Dis 2006;33(8):502–8.
81. Silverberg MJ, Thorsen P, Lindeberg H, et al. Condyloma in pregnancy is strongly predictive of juvenile-onset recurrent respiratory papillomatosis. Obstet Gynecol 2003;101(4):645–52.
82. Kashima HK, Shah F, Lyles A, et al. A comparison of risk factors in juvenile-onset and adult-onset recurrent respiratory papillomatosis. Laryngoscope 1992; 102(1):9–13.
83. Shah KV, Stern WF, Shah FK, et al. Risk factors for juvenile onset recurrent respiratory papillomatosis. Pediatr Infect Dis J 1998;17(5):372–6.
84. Rombaldi RL, Serafini EP, Mandelli J, et al. Transplacental transmission of human papillomavirus. Virol J 2008;5:106.
85. Winckworth LC, Nichol R. Question 2: do caesarean sections reduce the maternal-fetal transmission rate of human papillomavirus infection? Arch Dis Child 2010;95(1):70–3.

86. Puranen MH, Yliskoski MH, Saarikoski SV, et al. Exposure of an infant to cervical human papillomavirus infection of the mother is common. Am J Obstet Gynecol 1997;176(5):1039–45.

87. Bandyopadhyay S, Sen S, Majumdar L, et al. Human papillomavirus infection among Indian mothers and their infants. Asian Pac J Cancer Prev 2003;4(3): 179–84.

88. Smith EM, Ritchie JM, Yankowitz J, et al. Human papillomavirus prevalence and types in newborns and parents: concordance and modes of transmission. Sex Transm Dis 2004;31(1):57–62.

89. Wang X, Zhu Q, Rao H. Maternal-fetal transmission of human papillomavirus. Chin Med J (Engl) 1998;111(8):726–7.

90. Tseng CJ, Liang CC, Soong YK, et al. Perinatal transmission of human papillomavirus in infants: relationship between infection rate and mode of delivery. Obstet Gynecol 1998;91(1):92–6.

91. Tenti P, Zappatore R, Migliora P, et al. Perinatal transmission of human papillomavirus from gravidas with latent infections. Obstet Gynecol 1999;93(4):475–9.

92. Villa LL, Costa RL, Petta CA, et al. Prophylactic quadrivalent human papillomavirus (types 6, 11, 16, and 18) L1 virus-like particle vaccine in young women: a randomised double-blind placebo-controlled multicentre phase II efficacy trial. Lancet Oncol 2005;6(5):271–8.

93. Markowitz LE, Dunne EF, Saraiya M, et al. Quadrivalent human papillomavirus vaccine: recommendations of the Advisory Committee on Immunization Practices (ACIP). MMWR Recomm Rep 2007;56(RR-2):1–24.

94. Dallard C. Legislating against arousal: the growing divide between federal policy and teenage sexual behavior. Gutmacher Policy Rev 2006;9:12–6.

95. May J. HPV vaccination - a paradigm shift in public health. Aust Fam Physician 2007;36(3):106–11.

96. Gallagher TQ, Derkay CS. Recurrent respiratory papillomatosis: update 2008. Curr Opin Otolaryngol Head Neck Surg 2008;16(6):536–42.

97. Schaffer A, Brotherton J, Booy R. Do human papillomavirus vaccines have any role in newborns and the prevention of recurrent respiratory papillomatosis in children? J Paediatr Child Health 2007;43(9):579–80.

98. Kashima H, Mounts P, Leventhal B, et al. Sites of predilection in recurrent respiratory papillomatosis. Ann Otol Rhinol Laryngol 1993;102(8 Pt 1):580–3.

99. Silverberg MJ, Thorsen P, Lindeberg H, et al. Clinical course of recurrent respiratory papillomatosis in Danish children. Arch Otolaryngol Head Neck Surg 2004;130(6):711–6.

100. Wetmore RF, Muntz HR, McGill TJI. Pediatric otolaryngology: principles and practice pathways. New York: Thieme; 2000.

101. Cohn AM, Kos JT, Taber LH, et al. Recurring laryngeal papilloma. Am J Otolaryngol 1981;2(2):129–32.

102. Schraff S, Derkay CS, Burke B, et al. American Society of Pediatric Otolaryngology members' experience with recurrent respiratory papillomatosis and the use of adjuvant therapy. Arch Otolaryngol Head Neck Surg 2004;130(9):1039–42.

103. Xue Q, Wang J. Recurrent respiratory papillomatosis arising in trachea not affecting larynx. Intern Med 2010;49(15):1649–51.

104. Katsenos S, Becker HD. Recurrent respiratory papillomatosis: a rare chronic disease, difficult to treat, with potential to lung cancer transformation: apropos of two cases and a brief literature review. Case Rep Oncol 2011;4(1):162–71.

105. Cook JR, Hill DA, Humphrey PA, et al. Squamous cell carcinoma arising in recurrent respiratory papillomatosis with pulmonary involvement: emerging common

pattern of clinical features and human papillomavirus serotype association. Mod Pathol 2000;13(8):914–8.

106. Derkay CS, Malis DJ, Zalzal G, et al. A staging system for assessing severity of disease and response to therapy in recurrent respiratory papillomatosis. Laryngoscope 1998;108(6):935–7.

107. Derkay CS, Hester RP, Burke B, et al. Analysis of a staging assessment system for prediction of surgical interval in recurrent respiratory papillomatosis. Int J Pediatr Otorhinolaryngol 2004;68(12):1493–8.

108. Cole RR, Myer CM III, Cotton RT. Tracheotomy in children with recurrent respiratory papillomatosis. Head Neck 1989;11(3):226–30.

109. Healy GB, Gelber RD, Trowbridge AL, et al. Treatment of recurrent respiratory papillomatosis with human leukocyte interferon. Results of a multicenter randomized clinical trial. N Engl J Med 1988;319(7):401–7.

110. Leventhal BG, Kashima HK, Mounts P, et al. Long-term response of recurrent respiratory papillomatosis to treatment with lymphoblastoid interferon alfa-N1. Papilloma Study Group. N Engl J Med 1991;325(9):613–7.

111. Gerein V, Rastorguev E, Gerein J, et al. Use of interferon-alpha in recurrent respiratory papillomatosis: 20-year follow-up. Ann Otol Rhinol Laryngol 2005; 114(6):463–71.

112. Morrison GA, Kotecha B, Evans JN. Ribavirin treatment for juvenile respiratory papillomatosis. J Laryngol Otol 1993;107(5):423–6.

113. Shehab N, Sweet BV, Hogikyan ND. Cidofovir for the treatment of recurrent respiratory papillomatosis: a review of the literature. Pharmacotherapy 2005; 25(7):977–89.

114. Ksiazek J, Prager JD, Sun GH, et al. Inhaled cidofovir as an adjuvant therapy for recurrent respiratory papillomatosis. Otolaryngol Head Neck Surg 2011;144(4): 639–41.

115. Pransky SM, Albright JT, Magit AE. Long-term follow-up of pediatric recurrent respiratory papillomatosis managed with intralesional cidofovir. Laryngoscope 2003;113(9):1583–7.

116. Milczuk HA. Intralesional cidofovir for the treatment of severe juvenile recurrent respiratory papillomatosis: long-term results in 4 children. Otolaryngol Head Neck Surg 2003;128(6):788–94.

117. Akst LM, Lee W, Discolo C, et al. Stepped-dose protocol of cidofovir therapy in recurrent respiratory papillomatosis in children. Arch Otolaryngol Head Neck Surg 2003;129(8):841–6.

118. Lee AS, Rosen CA. Efficacy of cidofovir injection for the treatment of recurrent respiratory papillomatosis. J Voice 2004;18(4):551–6.

119. Peyton SW, Wiatrak B. Is cidofovir a useful adjunctive therapy for recurrent respiratory papillomatosis in children? Int J Pediatr Otorhinolaryngol 2004; 68(4):413–8.

120. Mandell DL, Arjmand EM, Kay DJ, et al. Intralesional cidofovir for pediatric recurrent respiratory papillomatosis. Arch Otolaryngol Head Neck Surg 2004; 130(11):1319–23.

121. Naiman AN, Ceruse P, Coulombeau B, et al. Intralesional cidofovir and surgical excision for laryngeal papillomatosis. Laryngoscope 2003;113(12):2174–81.

122. Goon P, Sonnex C, Jani P, et al. Recurrent respiratory papillomatosis: an overview of current thinking and treatment. Eur Arch Otorhinolaryngol 2008;265(2): 147–51.

123. Wutzler P, Thust R. Genetic risks of antiviral nucleoside analogues–a survey. Antiviral Res 2001;49(2):55–74.

124. Chadha NK, James AL. Antiviral agents for the treatment of recurrent respiratory papillomatosis: a systematic review of the English-language literature. Otolaryngol Head Neck Surg 2007;136(6):863–9.
125. Rosen CA, Bryson PC. Indole-3-carbinol for recurrent respiratory papillomatosis: long-term results. J Voice 2004;18(2):248–53.
126. Derkay CS, Smith RJ, McClay J, et al. HspE7 treatment of pediatric recurrent respiratory papillomatosis: final results of an open-label trial. Ann Otol Rhinol Laryngol 2005;114(9):730–7.
127. Pashley NR. Can mumps vaccine induce remission in recurrent respiratory papilloma? Arch Otolaryngol Head Neck Surg 2002;128(7):783–6.
128. Lieu JE, Molter DW. Another potential adjuvant therapy for recurrent respiratory papillomatosis. Arch Otolaryngol Head Neck Surg 2002;128(7):787–8.
129. Dolmans DE, Fukumura D, Jain RK. Photodynamic therapy for cancer. Nat Rev Cancer 2003;3(5):380–7.
130. Dougherty TJ, Gomer CJ, Henderson BW, et al. Photodynamic therapy. J Natl Cancer Inst 1998;90(12):889–905.
131. Shikowitz MJ, Abramson AL, Steinberg BM, et al. Clinical trial of photodynamic therapy with meso-tetra (hydroxyphenyl) chlorin for respiratory papillomatosis. Arch Otolaryngol Head Neck Surg 2005;131(2):99–105.
132. Lee RG, Vecchiotti MA, Heaphy J, et al. Photodynamic therapy of cottontail rabbit papillomavirus-induced papillomas in a severe combined immunodeficient mouse xenograft system. Laryngoscope 2010;120(3):618–24.
133. Abramson AL, Shikowitz MJ, Mullooly VM, et al. Clinical effects of photodynamic therapy on recurrent laryngeal papillomas. Arch Otolaryngol Head Neck Surg 1992;118(1):25–9.
134. Abramson AL, Shikowitz MJ, Mullooly VM, et al. Variable light-dose effect on photodynamic therapy for laryngeal papillomas. Arch Otolaryngol Head Neck Surg 1994;120(8):852–5.
135. Borkowski G, Sommer P, Stark T, et al. Recurrent respiratory papillomatosis associated with gastroesophageal reflux disease in children. Eur Arch Otorhinolaryngol 1999;256(7):370–2.
136. Harcourt JP, Worley G, Leighton SE. Cimetidine treatment for recurrent respiratory papillomatosis. Int J Pediatr Otorhinolaryngol 1999;51(2):109–13.
137. McKenna M, Brodsky L. Extraesophageal acid reflux and recurrent respiratory papilloma in children. Int J Pediatr Otorhinolaryngol 2005;69(5):597–605.
138. Holland BW, Koufman JA, Postma GN, et al. Laryngopharyngeal reflux and laryngeal web formation in patients with pediatric recurrent respiratory papillomas. Laryngoscope 2002;112(11):1926–9.

Pierre Robin Sequence

Evaluation, Management, Indications for Surgery, and Pitfalls

Andrew R. Scott, MD[a,*], Robert J. Tibesar, MD[b,c],
James D. Sidman, MD[b,c]

KEYWORDS

- Cleft palate • Micrognathia • Glossoptosis • Pediatric sleep apnea
- Mandibular distraction osteogenesis • Tongue-lip adhesion • Pierre Robin Sequence

KEY POINTS

- Pierre Robin Sequence (PRS) is a triad of micrognathia, glossoptosis, and cleft palate, which may occur as isolated findings in an otherwise normal child or be associated with additional syndromic features.
- Children with PRS may exhibit varying degrees of upper airway obstruction.
- Management of upper airway obstruction is best approached conservatively, using nonoperative interventions first.
- The majority of infants are stabilized by nonsurgical measures.
- Children with neurologic deficits at risk for chronic aspiration are better served by traditional surgical interventions such as tracheotomy and gastrostomy-tube placement.
- Mandibular distraction osteogenesis is the only surgical technique that directly addresses the underlying cause of upper airway obstruction in PRS without compromising feeding. It offers results that persist through early childhood.
- Mandibular distraction procedure mandates specialized training.
- Complications of neonatal mandibular distraction osteogenesis:

The authors have no financial interests to disclose.
Dr James Sidman is a paid consultant for Medtronic, Inc.
Conflict of interest: None.
[a] Department of Otolaryngology – Head & Neck Surgery, Floating Hospital for Children – Tufts Medical Center, Tufts University School of Medicine, Box 850, 800 Washington Street, Boston, MA 02111, USA; [b] Pediatric ENT Associates, Children's Specialty Center, Children's Hospitals and Clinics of Minnesota, 2530 Chicago Avenue South, Suite 450, Minneapolis, MN 55404, USA; [c] Department of Otolaryngology, University of Minnesota Medical School, Phillips Wangensteen Building, 516 Delaware Street SE, Suite 8A, Minneapolis, MN 55455, USA
* Corresponding author.
E-mail address: ascott@tuftsmedicalcenter.org

Short Term	Long Term
Infection	Tooth loss
Hardware failure	Scarring
Bone resorption and regression	Asymmetry
Nonunion	Corrective orthodontics
Facial nerve injury	Additional surgeries
Open-bite deformity	

Much has been written about airway interventions in children with Pierre Robin Sequence (PRS), with many investigators from a variety of disciplines advocating any number of methods used to manage the problem. This article seeks to review the various methods of treating airway obstruction and feeding difficulty in infants with PRS, and highlights the benefits and limitations of early mandibular distraction osteogenesis, particularly as a way of managing both airway obstruction and feeding difficulty in these children.

PRS was first described in 1923 by Pierre Robin, a French stomatologist, as a diad of micrognathia and glossoptosis.[1] In 1934 he revised the definition to include a triad of micrognathia, glossoptosis, and a U-shaped cleft palate.[2] It is not a syndrome in itself, but rather a sequence in which multiple secondary anomalies are derived from a single anomaly, and affects approximately 1 in 8500 births. The prevailing hypothesis implicates hypoplasia of the mandible (either from a primary growth disturbance or from hyperflexion of the neck) before 9 weeks in utero as the inciting factor. The small jaw positions the tongue posteriorly and superiorly where it lies between the 2 palatal shelves, physically preventing their fusion, which normally occurs between the 8th and 10th weeks of gestation. It is this mechanical disruption of palatal closure and not a primary molecular or genetic factor that leads to the palatal cleft. Many newborns with PRS have upper airway obstruction and exhibit varying degrees of respiratory distress, which may require intervention. In addition, children may struggle with oral feeding, owing to the difficulty in coordinating breathing and swallowing in the context of tongue-base obstruction and a cleft palate.

DIAGNOSIS OF PIERRE ROBIN SEQUENCE

The diagnosis of PRS is typically made at birth. With improvements in prenatal imaging including high-resolution ultrasonography, micrognathia is now being diagnosed as early as the second trimester of pregnancy. In light of this there has been an attempt to standardize mandibular measurements on ultrasonography, including comparison with other cephalometric proportions[3,4] and creation of a mandibular index, which takes into account the anterior/posterior dimension of the mandible as it relates to the biparietal diameter of the fetus.[5] In practice, however, these measurements are rarely used, and micrognathia is often a relatively subjective call by the examining maternal fetal medicine physician. Inspection of the mandible is possible with ultrasonography, but evaluation of the tongue and palate is less reliable. Although the diagnosis of micrognathia can be made in utero, confirmation of the complete triad of PRS before delivery is usually not possible.

Physical Examination

At birth, the micrognathia is the most striking feature. This trait is characterized by a small and retrusive mandible in which the mandibular alveolus is significantly posterior to the maxillary alveolus. Examination of the oral cavity reveals posterior and superior positioning of the tongue (**Fig. 1**). Palatal examination will show a U-shaped cleft palate involving the soft palate and posterior hard palate; the alveolus is spared. Often the tongue is positioned within the palatal cleft itself, especially when the child is supine.

Some infants exhibit minimal respiratory symptoms at birth whereas others have significant airway obstruction, with stertor, retractions, and even cyanosis. These symptoms are usually worse when the child is lying supine, owing to gravity-dependent tongue-base obstruction, which occurs at the level of the oropharynx.

PRS may be the only abnormality noted on newborn examination, or may be noted as part of several dysmorphic features owing to a unifying, syndromic diagnosis. For this reason, some children with PRS are robust and vigorous, whereas others may have significant hypotonia (due to underlying neurologic impairment) or worrisome cyanosis (due to structural heart disease, for example). Examination of the ears, eyes, heart, and extremities may point toward a diagnosis of Nagar, Stickler, or veloc-ardiofacial syndrome, to name a few. For this reason a full evaluation by a geneticist is helpful for categorizing infants with PRS into those with isolated findings and those with additional syndromic features. Children with neurologic impairment are at a higher risk than their peers with isolated PRS of requiring surgical intervention for airway distress.[6]

Endoscopic Examination

Additional evaluation of the airway obstruction with fiberoptic nasal laryngoscopy is useful. Endoscopic examination usually confirms tongue-base obstruction and may identify synchronous airway lesions such as laryngomalacia. Additional causes of upper airway obstruction have been described in PRS, including lateral pharyngeal wall motion and pharyngeal narrowing without glossoptosis.[7] While most children with PRS suffer from obstruction related to glossoptosis, indentifying these other variants is essential, as choosing the appropriate airway intervention requires accurate identification of the site of obstruction. For this reason not all children with PRS are effectively managed with interventions that target tongue-base obstruction alone.

Polysomnography

Quantifying the degree of respiratory compromise can be challenging. Polysomnography may be used to document the extent of airway obstruction and rule out any potential aspect of central apnea contributing to the infant's respiratory distress. Often polysomnography is not necessary or even possible, for that matter, as many children

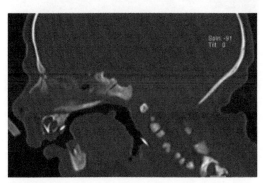

Fig. 1. Computed tomography scan of a child with Pierre Robin Sequence. Even with the child nasotracheally intubated, glossoptosis is evident.

have life-threatening airway obstruction when awake, obviating evaluation when they are unconscious.

Laboratory Studies

Laboratory studies may be used to support the diagnosis of chronic airway obstruction in those children without frank respiratory failure. Serial capillary blood gases may be used to document a trend of elevated or increasing carbon dioxide levels, thus suggesting chronic hypoventilation or worsening carbon dioxide retention.

All children with PRS should be observed in a monitored setting such as the neonatal intensive care unit, where continuous-pulse oximetry and cardiac monitoring are used.

INITIAL AIRWAY MANAGEMENT FOR MICROGNATHIA

There is a variety of options available for airway management in the micrognathic child. Some children require no intervention whatsoever. However, many infants do display signs of upper airway obstruction, and when this occurs it is most reasonable to begin with the most conservative measures. The authors' philosophy is to start with side and prone positioning. If the problem persists, placement of a nasopharyngeal airway can be helpful in both bypassing the tongue-base obstruction and in breaking the seal made between the oropharyngeal tongue and the posterior pharyngeal wall (**Fig. 2**). A variety of custom oral appliances may also be fashioned for the purpose of relieving obstruction, and the literature is replete with reports on institutional experiences with these devices.[8–10] Other investigators have described success at using customized endotracheal tubes to relieve obstruction.[11]

SURGICAL INTERVENTIONS FOR UPPER AIRWAY OBSTRUCTION

Nonsurgical management of upper airway obstruction in children with PRS is not only possible; it is preferable. Retrospective reviews examining airway interventions in infants with PRS consistently demonstrate that most children may be successfully managed nonoperatively.[6,12–16] Nevertheless, some patients are unable to tolerate oropharyngeal stents or nasopharyngeal airways; management of these devices may prove overwhelming to providers and parents alike.

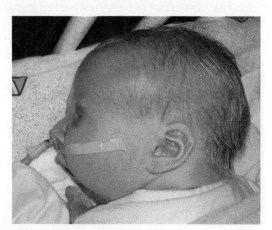

Fig. 2. A child with Pierre Robin Sequence and upper airway obstruction severe enough to merit intervention with a nasopharyngeal airway.

SURGICAL INTERVENTIONS TO ADDRESS TONGUE-BASE OBSTRUCTION IN PRS
Tongue-Lip Adhesion

A variety of glossopexy procedures have been described including tongue-lip adhesion (TLA), which may be performed with or without subperiosteal release of the floor of mouth and circum-mandibular suturing.[17] In one popular technique, the genioglossus musculature is released from the mandible and the circum-mandibular suture technique is used to anchor the tongue-base to the inferior alveolus. Mucosal flaps, which were raised from the ventral tongue and the ends of the gingivolabial sulcus are then brought together to complete the adhesion (**Fig. 3**).[17] The adhesion is maintained throughout the first year of life and is typically taken down at the time of palate repair, which takes place at approximately age 9 to 12 months. Although the success rate of this technique at managing airway obstruction is as high as 89% in select patients,[18] tethering the mobile tongue anteriorly tends to exacerbate the child's underlying dysphagia, increasing the likelihood of requiring a prolonged period of enteral feeding supplementation via nasogastric catheter or gastrostomy tube.[12,13,18] In a recent review of a single institution's experience with TLA, 54% of children in whom airway obstruction was successfully managed by this procedure required gastrostomy-tube placement to assure adequate nutritional intake.[18] In 1998, a survey of airway surgeons at pediatric centers caring for children with PRS suggested that more than 80% of institutions have abandoned this technique.[19] However. the minority of centers who still use TLA believe it is a worthwhile intervention and are satisfied with their results.[13,18] Advocates cite the relative simplicity of the procedure, lack of long-term scarring, avoidance of potential nerve or tooth injury, and lack of specialized equipment as major advantages of the TLA technique over more complex and expensive orthognathic procedures. Critics of the technique cite variable results and significant postoperative dysphagia requiring prolonged nasogastric or gastrostomy-tube feeding. For this reason the authors believe that those children who can be stabilized with TLA are likely the same group of patients successfully managed with nasopharyngeal airways with or without nasogastric feeding.

Tracheotomy

Traditional algorithms for airway management in children with PRS point to the use of tracheotomy as a final backup for children who fail TLA, as it is considered the

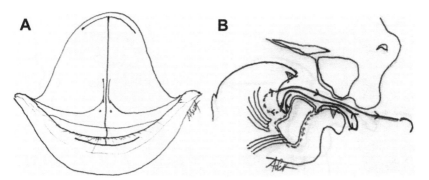

Fig. 3. (*A*) Mirror-image "T" incisions used during tongue-lip adhesion. (*B*) Diagrammatic representation of circum-mandibular and tongue-base suturing technique as described by Argamasso.[17]

definitive technique for securing a stable airway in any patient with upper airway obstruction. Although a tracheotomy will reliably and successfully bypass the site of tongue-base obstruction, it is a procedure with potential long-term morbidity and mortality.[20,21] Complications associated with tracheotomy include:

- Sudden airway obstruction from accidental decannulation or mucous plugging
- Airway infections
- Bleeding
- Stomal maintenance problems
- Tracheal stenosis
- Inhibition of proper speech and swallowing development.

Furthermore, children with tracheotomies require skilled nursing care at home and in their educational facilities, along with monitoring and suction equipment, among other resources. Nevertheless, in a survey of otolaryngologists at large fellowship training centers, 52% chose tracheotomy as the treatment of choice for airway management in children with PRS.[19]

Mandibular Distraction Osteogenesis

Another option for the management of airway obstruction in the neonatal period is mandibular distraction osteogenesis (MDO). This technique, in which the mandible is slowly advanced after an initial osteotomy, relieves supraglottic airway obstruction by bringing the tongue base forward (**Fig. 4**). This surgery is now widely used across the United States for select children with micrognathia and severe airway obstruction as an alternative to tracheotomy. This technique is gaining wider acceptance among plastic craniofacial surgeons and pediatric otolaryngologists alike, as feeding outcomes in general are more favorable than those observed with TLA, allowing children to avoid both a tracheotomy and a gastrostomy tube in most cases.[22–25] The specifics of patient selection, operative technique, and protocol for postoperative

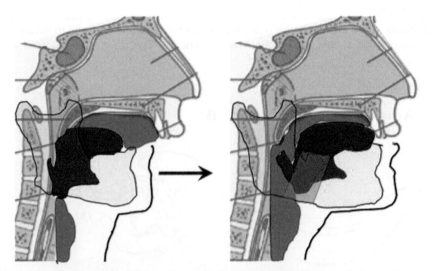

Fig. 4. The concept behind bilateral mandibular distraction osteogenesis, in which supraglottic tongue-base obstruction is relieved by anterior advancement of the hypoplastic mandible.

distraction are described later in this article. Potential early and long-term complications are also discussed.

FEEDING INTERVENTIONS IN CHILDREN WITH PRS

In addition to the airway problems, many patients with PRS are not able to sufficiently feed orally. Their airway obstruction prevents a normal swallow and they cannot maintain an adequate caloric intake, often causing these children to require supplemental enteric feeding via nasogastric catheter.[12,13] Furthermore, gastrostomy-tube placement sometimes follows initial attempts at nasogastric feeding, owing to frequent displacement and intermittent occlusion of nasoenteric feeding catheters.

Institutional Reviews

Retrospective institutional reviews have shown varying rates of gastrostomy-tube placement in children with PRS, with the need for gastrostomy-tube placement potentially influenced by the management strategy used for addressing the airway obstruction in these infants.

- For example, one published series of 115 PRS infants from 2 institutions that manage airway obstruction with TLA or tracheotomy had an overall gastrostomy-tube placement rate of 41% for nonsyndromic children.[12]
- A related case series of 53 infants with PRS managed with TLA showed a gastrostomy placement rate of 38% for nonsyndromic children and upwards of 83% for syndromic PRS infants.[18]
- A second institutional review of 29 children with airway obstruction severe enough to merit TLA showed a preoperative enteral feeding rate of 93% and a postoperative rate of 72%, 27% requiring supplementation beyond 6 months after the procedure.[13]
- Conversely, a review of 67 infants with PRS from a third institution that performs early MDO or tracheotomy demonstrated an overall gastrostomy placement rate of 10% for nonsyndromic PRS children and as high as 75% for syndromic infants.[23] Further classifications of these subjects showed that of 14 nonsyndromic PRS children managed with MDO, none of them came to require a gastrostomy tube. However, upwards of 88% of syndromic patients managed with early MDO ultimately came to require gastrostomy.[23]

These findings highlight the universally accepted understanding that syndromic PRS children tend to fare worse than those with the isolated disorder.[14–16] It seems that the greatest differences in results between groups that manage airway obstruction with TLA versus those that use MDO are observed in feeding outcomes. These differences are most striking in the nonsyndromic PRS population (**Fig. 5; Tables 1 and 2**).[6,12,18,23,24]

EVIDENCE SUPPORTING MANDIBULAR DISTRACTION OSTEOGENESIS

MDO is a technique in which the mandible is gradually lengthened after an initial osteotomy. Following a short latency period, distraction begins at a slow, steady rate. During this phase, bone segments are separated by small increments and induction of new bone formation takes place in the gap. After the desired lengthening has been achieved, a consolidation period ensues in which the bone segments are held securely in their advanced position. The regenerate of immature bone remodels and matures during this 4- to 6-week time frame, after which the distraction hardware is

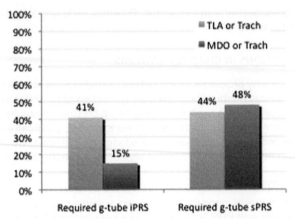

Fig. 5. A comparison of feeding outcomes between institutions that use differing strategies for operatively managing airway obstruction in Pierre Robin Sequence. Note the difference in the rate of g-tube placement for nonsyndromic children versus the nearly identical rate of enteral feeding in syndromic children. g-tube, gastrostomy tube; iPRS, isolated Pierre Robin Sequence; MDO, mandibular distraction osteogenesis; sPRS, syndromic Pierre Robin Sequence; TLA, tongue-lip adhesion; Trach, tracheotomy.

removed. Because distraction proceeds at a slow pace, related muscles, blood vessels, nerves, skin, and mucosa are also elongated during the process. This concomitant expansion of soft tissue is one of the main advantages of MDO (**Fig. 6**).

- McCarthy was the first to report on use of mandibular distraction in pediatric patients with micrognathia.[25]
- Cohen and colleagues[26] described the use of bilateral MDO to treat obstructive sleep apnea in children with craniofacial anomalies in 1998, reporting on use of the technique in child as young as 14 weeks of age.
- In 2001, Denny and colleagues[27] and Sidman and colleagues[28] published additional reports documenting the use of bilateral MDO for the primary purpose of relieving upper airway obstruction.
- Over the past decade numerous investigators have published personal series of pediatric MDO, highlighting various techniques and reporting on early results.

Several centers now use the technique of bilateral MDO to improve airway obstruction and feeding difficulties in infants and newborns.[27–29] Because this is still a relatively new practice, critics of MDO have noted that long-term morbidity from this invasive procedure is still unknown.[12,13,18] There are growing data, however, on the long-term results following early bilateral MDO for relief of upper airway obstruction.[22,24,25,29–33] Although these studies are limited in their sample size, the nature and severity of long-term outcomes and complication rates for bilateral MDO in this age group are similar to those seen in established larger series of adolescent and adult patients.[34,35]

A recent report from our institution examined the long-term outcomes of 19 children younger than 3 months with PRS who underwent bilateral MDO as a means of avoiding tracheotomy when conservative management with positioning and nasopharyngeal airway intervention failed.[23] TLA was not used in this cohort. Mandibular distraction allowed for avoidance of tracheotomy in all children with isolated PRS and syndromic PRS without neurologic deficits. Of those children with syndromic PRS and neurologic

Table 1
Comparison of retrospective studies examining airway interventions and outcomes from 4 institutions

Study	Year	Subjects (N)	iPRS (n)	sPRS (n)	Type of Intervention	Rate of Operative Intervention Overall (%)	Rate of Intervention iPRS (%)	Rate of Intervention sPRS (%)	Required g-tube iPRS (%)	Required g-tube sPRS (%)
Kirschner et al[13]	2003	107	N/A	N/A	TLA or Trach	31	N/A	N/A	N/A	N/A
Evans et al[12]	2006	115	63	52	TLA or Trach	44	N/A	N/A	41	44
Meyer et al[6]	2008	74	53	21	MDO or Trach	32	30	38	15	48

Abbreviations: g-tube, gastrostomy tube; iPRS, isolated Pierre Robin Sequence; MDO, mandibular distraction osteogenesis; N/A, no data available; sPRS, syndromic Pierre Robin Sequence; TLA, tongue–lip adhesion; Trach, tracheotomy.

Table 2
Comparison of two recent retrospective studies, one examining outcomes following tongue-lip adhesion and the other following early mandibular distraction

Study	Year	Subjects (N)	iPRS (n)	sPRS (n)	Intervention	Required Tracheotomy iPRS (%)	Required Tracheotomy sPRS Without Neurologic Impairment (%)	Required Tracheotomy sPRS With Neurologic Impairment (%)	Required g-tube iPRS (%)	Required g-tube sPRS (%)
Rogers et al[18]	2011	53	29	24	TLA	0	7	50	38	83
Scott et al[24]	2011	19	14	5	MDO	0	0	50	7	40

Abbreviations: g-tube, gastrostomy tube; iPRS, isolated Pierre Robin Sequence; MDO, mandibular distraction osteogenesis; sPRS, syndromic Pierre Robin Sequence; TLA, tongue-lip adhesion.

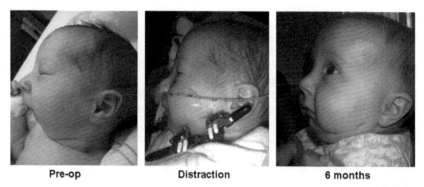

| Pre-op | Distraction | 6 months |

Fig. 6. Short-term results following bilateral mandibular distraction osteogenesis in an infant with isolated Pierre Robin Sequence who failed nonoperative management of airway obstruction and feeding difficulty.

impairment, 50% failed airway management with MDO and underwent subsequent tracheotomy. These outcomes mirror those reported by Rogers and colleagues[18] in 2011 in regard of their success with TLA (**Fig. 7**; see **Table 2**).

In contrast to the TLA series, children who underwent MDO had a lower rate of gastrostomy-tube placement overall, most evident in the isolated PRS group (see **Fig. 5**). The MDO cohort was relatively small, which limits the statistical impact of the case series; however, this trend is borne out in larger studies comparing overall rates of gastrostomy-tube placement between institutions operatively managing PRS with TLA or tracheotomy versus those who use MDO or tracheotomy (see **Table 1**).[6,12] The small sample size of the series of Scott and colleagues[24] is countered by its considerable length of follow-up (average 5.6 years).

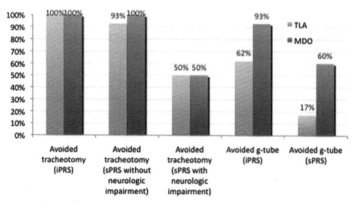

Fig. 7. A comparison of airway and feeding outcomes for tongue-lip adhesion versus mandibular distraction based on 2 retrospective studies.[18,24] Note the nearly identical airway outcomes compared with the feeding outcomes for the 2 interventions. g-tube, gastrostomy tube; iPRS, isolated Pierre Robin Sequence; MDO, mandibular distraction osteogenesis; sPRS, syndromic Pierre Robin Sequence; TLA, tongue-lip adhesion.

Complications of MDO

- Damage to the developing molars was the most common complication and occurred in 21% of patients.
- Mandibular growth disturbance was not as significant, with only one child requiring a secondary procedure.
- External scarring was an issue, with the surgeon recommending scar revision on one or both sides in 15% of children; interestingly none of the parents felt it was necessary.
- Injury to the marginal mandibular branch of the facial nerve occurred in 15% of patients and was usually temporary.
- Regarding inferior alveolar nerve damage, direct testing of sensation in the mental nerve distribution in these children did not reveal any subjective deficits; objective testing was never performed.[24]

Critics of MDO point to the risks of complications noted here and also to the cost of the distraction devices and paucity of surgeons trained in the technique. Supporters of MDO will point to similar airway outcomes to those of TLA but an overall lower gastrostomy placement rate. This outcome is probably due to the fact that TLA is a finite intervention with the goal of serving as a temporizing measure, rather than a definitive procedure that ameliorates both breathing and feeding difficulties. Both interventions are proven and valid techniques for addressing airway obstruction in select infants with PRS, and providers will have to judge for themselves as to whether the potential increased risks of early MDO are justified in avoiding a prolonged need to enteral feeding in the first year of life and subsequent potential morbidities of oral aversion, social issues, stomal maintenance, and scarring when gastrostomy tubes are used.

PEARLS & PITFALLS: *It remains of vital importance to identify those children with PRS who are good candidates for TLA and MDO and those who are not. Certain subsets of syndromic PRS infants have a high likelihood of TLA or MDO failure, and would therefore benefit from upfront tracheotomy and gastrostomy-tube placement.*[6,12,13,18,25]

Predictive Testing for Surgery Outcome

Several studies have sought to identify preoperative characteristics in infants with PRS that could be used to predict which patients will fail. Two studies in 2011 described factors that were predictive of poor airway outcomes following TLA and MDO with eventual need for salvage tracheotomy.

Rogers and colleagues[18] developed the GILLS score, which can be used to identify those patients with PRS who have a high likelihood of failing TLA. The acronym GILLS was created to serve as a 5-point scale, with GILLS scores of 3 or more suggestive of a failure rate above 40%:

Gastroesophageal reflux
Intubation preoperatively
Late operation (older than age 2 weeks)
Low birth weight (<2500 g)
Syndromic diagnosis.

A smaller study involving long-term follow-up of children with PRS who underwent early MDO (younger than 3 months) showed a trend toward poor outcomes (need for eventual tracheotomy and/or gastrostomy, among other unfavorable results) in syndromic PRS infants who also had neurologic impairment such as seizures, hypotonia, and chronic aspiration.[24]

The overarching theme of both of these studies suggests that nonsyndromic PRS children tend to have favorable airway outcomes following TLA or MDO, and that certain syndromic children without neurocognitive comorbidities (eg, Stickler syndrome) fare equally as well as their nonsyndromic peers.[13,18,24] The exception to this may lie in syndromic children with primary growth disturbances of the mandible such as those with oculo-auricular-vertebral, Treacher-Collins, or Nager syndrome, for example. In these patients there is an underlying disturbance in the growth center below the mandibular condyle which may limit, if not prevent, growth of the jaw, even after a "head start" offered by early mandibular distraction. In addition, children with absent mandibular condyles, absent coronoid process, and a poorly defined glenoid fossa (Pruzansky Grade 3)[36] are not ideally suited for early distraction (**Fig. 8**).[37] In these infants, the posterior mandibular segment may not engage properly against the skull base, allowing seemingly infinite posterior movement into the soft tissue of the mastoid area, thus preventing effective anterior advancement of the mandible with distraction of the mobile segments. The authors have chosen to treat this subset of children with upfront tracheotomy followed by costal cartilage grafting and creation of a pseudarthrosis at the temporomandibular joint site later in childhood. Following these procedures, the jaw is advanced through distraction of the grafted rib segment.

*PEARLS & PITFALLS: **Many investigators have noted that children with PRS who are also neurologically impaired are at risk for airway compromise from factors that are independent of their glossoptosis.**[13–16,18,24]*

For this reason, addressing tongue-base obstruction with glossopexy or distraction alone in this subset of syndromic PRS is not appropriate, as these surgical interventions do not treat coexisting hypotonia, poor coordination, or chronic aspiration. For children with these comorbidities, tracheotomy and gastrostomy-tube placement allows for bypass of any and all sites of upper airway obstruction, improved pulmonary toilet, and maintenance of enteral nutrition. Treating neurologically impaired children with TLA or MDO incurs additional costs and avoidable surgical risks related to such operative interventions.

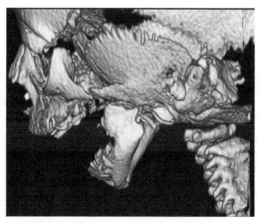

Fig. 8. Abnormal development of the temporomandibular joint as demonstrated on a computed tomography scan of a newborn with syndromic Pierre Robin Sequence.

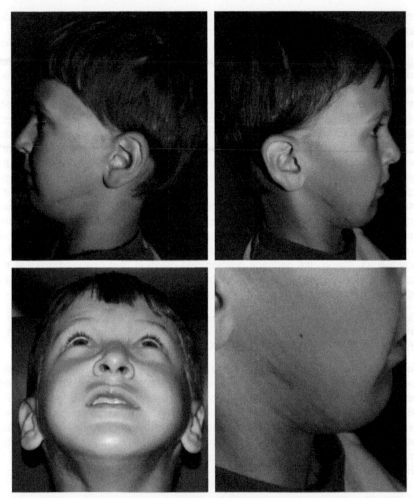

Fig. 9. Long-term results following neonatal mandibular distraction osteogenesis as seen in this 7-year-old boy. Scars are evident but not bothersome to the patient or the family, and scar revision has been deferred.

PEARLS & PITFALLS: A comment should be made about the potential pitfalls of the various surgical approaches to mandibular distraction in particular. Hardware may be placed through a transcervical or transoral approach with use of either external or buried hardware.

For neonatal distraction, most surgeons use an external approach with either external devices or buried hardware. The greatest benefit of using buried hardware is less external scarring. However, disadvantages include more significant operative dissection, greater potential for developing postoperative open-bite deformity (with use of linear, unidirectional devices), and a more invasive secondary operation for removal of the device that puts the facial nerve at risk for injury, especially during mobilization of the posterior hardware. The authors prefer to use multidirectional external distraction devices. Although placement of external k-wires leaves small scars on the cheeks in addition to the submandibular incisions (see **Fig. 6**), all incisions usually heal in a favorable manner over the long term[22] (**Fig. 9**) and minor scar revision is always possible. More importantly, the multidirectional distractors allow for instant correction of any developing open-bite deformity. Finally, the secondary operation for removal of these devices is simple and is performed under minimal sedation with mask ventilation. Percutaneous removal of k-wires alone obviates any repeat dissection, and there is no risk of nerve injury or additional scarring incurred by device removal.

REFERENCES

1. Robin P. La chute de la base de la langue considerée comme une nouvelle cause de gene dans la respiration nasopharyngienne. Bull Acad Med (Paris) 1923;89: 37–41.
2. Robin P. Glossoptosis due to atresia and hypotrophy of the mandible. Am J Dis Child 1934;48:541.
3. Malas MA, Ungör B, Tağil SM, et al. Determination of dimensions and angles of mandible in the fetal period. Surg Radiol Anat 2006;28(4):364–71.
4. Captier G, Faure JM, Bäumler M, et al. Prenatal assessment of the antero-posterior jaw relationship in human fetuses: from anatomical to ultrasound ceph-alometric analysis. Cleft Palate Craniofac J 2011;48(4):465–72.
5. Paladini D, Morra T, Teodoro A, et al. Objective diagnosis of micrognathia in the fetus: the jaw index. Obstet Gynecol 1999;93(3):382–6.
6. Meyer AC, Lidsky ME, Sampson DE, et al. Airway interventions in children with Pierre Robin Sequence. Otolaryngol Head Neck Surg 2008;138(6):782–7.
7. Sher AE. Mechanisms of airway obstruction in Robin sequence: implications for treatment. Cleft Palate Craniofac J 1992;29(3):224–31.
8. Pielou WD, Allen A. The use of an obturator in the management of the Pierre Robin syndrome. Dent Pract Dent Rec 1968;18(5):169–72.
9. Oktay H, Baydaş B, Ersöz M. Using a modified nutrition plate for early intervention in a newborn infant with Pierre Robin sequence: a case report. Cleft Palate Cra-niofac J 2006;43(3):370–3.
10. Bacher M, Sautermeister J, Urschitz MS, et al. An oral appliance with velar exten-sion for treatment of obstructive sleep apnea in infants with Pierre Robin sequence. Cleft Palate Craniofac J 2011;48(3):331–6.
11. Parhizkar N, Saltzman B, Grote K, et al. Nasopharyngeal airway for management of airway obstruction in infants with micrognathia. Cleft Palate Craniofac J 2011; 48(4):478–82.
12. Evans AK, Rahbar R, Rogers GF, et al. Robin sequence: a retrospective review of 115 patients. Int J Pediatr Otorhinolaryngol 2006;70(6):973–80.
13. Kirschner RE, Low DW, Randall P, et al. Surgical airway management in Pierre Robin sequence: is there a role for tongue-lip adhesion? Cleft Palate Craniofac J 2003;40(1):13–8.
14. Pashayan HM, Lewis MB. Clinical experience with the Robin sequence. Cleft Palate J 1984;21:270–6.
15. Caouette-Laberge L, Bayet B, Larocque Y. The Pierre Robin sequence: review of 125 cases and evolution of treatment modalities. Plast Reconstr Surg 1994;93: 934–42.
16. Tomaski SM, Zalzal GH, Saal HM. Airway obstruction in the Pierre Robin sequence. Laryngoscope 1995;105:111–4.
17. Argamaso RV. Glossopexy for upper airway obstruction in Robin sequence. Cleft Palate Craniofac J 1992;29:232–8.

18. Rogers GF, Murthy AS, LaBrie RA, et al. The GILLS score: part I. Patient selection for tongue-lip adhesion in Robin sequence. Plast Reconstr Surg 2011;128(1): 243–51.

19. Myer CM III, Reed JM, Cotton RT, et al. Airway management in Pierre Robin sequence. Otolaryngol Head Neck Surg 1998;118:630–5.

20. Gianoli GJ, Miller RH, Guarisco JL. Tracheotomy in the first year of life. Ann Otol Rhinol Laryngol 1990;99:896–901.

21. Wetmore RF, Handler SD, Potsic WP. Pediatric tracheostomy: experience during the past decade. Ann Otol Rhinol Laryngol 1982;91:628–32.

22. Tibesar RJ, Scott AR, McNamara C, et al. Distraction osteogenesis of the mandible for airway obstruction in children: long-term results. Otolaryngol Head Neck Surg 2010;143(1):90–6.

23. Lidsky ME, Lander TA, Sidman JD. Resolving feeding difficulties with early airway intervention in Pierre Robin Sequence. Laryngoscope 2008;118:120–3.

24. Scott AR, Tibesar RJ, Lander TA, et al. Mandibular distraction osteogenesis in infants younger than 3 months. Arch Facial Plast Surg 2011;13(3):173–9.

25. McCarthy JG, Schreiber J, Karp N, et al. Lengthening the human mandible by gradual distraction. Plast Reconstr Surg 1992;89:1.

26. Cohen SR, Simms C, Burstein FD. Mandibular distraction osteogenesis in treatment of upper airway obstruction in children with craniofacial deformities. Plast Reconstr Surg 1998;101:311.

27. Denny AD, Talisman R, Hanson PR, et al. Mandibular distraction osteogenesis in very young patients to correct airway obstruction. Plast Reconstr Surg 2001;108: 302–11.

28. Sidman JD, Sampson D, Templeton B. Distraction osteogenesis of the mandible for airway obstruction in children. Laryngoscope 2001;111:1137–46.

29. Lin SJ, Roy S, Patel PK. Distraction osteogenesis in the pediatric population. Otolaryngol Head Neck Surg 2007;137:233–8.

30. Kleine-Hakala M, Hukki J, Hurmerinta K. Effect of mandibular distraction osteogenesis on developing molars. Orthod Craniofac Res 2007;10:196–202.

31. McCarthy JG, Katzen JT, Hopper R, et al. The first decade of mandibular distraction: lessons we have learned. Plast Reconstr Surg 2002;110(7):1704–13.

32. Hollier LH, Kim J, Grayson B, et al. Mandibular growth after distraction in patients under 48 months of age. Plast Reconstr Surg 1999;103(5):1361–70.

33. Stelnicki EJ, Lin WY, Lee C, et al. Long-term outcome study of bilateral mandibular distraction: a comparison of Treacher Collins and Nager syndromes to other types of micrognathia. Plast Reconstr Surg 2002;109(6):1819–25 [discussion: 1826–7].

34. van Strijen PJ, Breuning KH, Becking AG, et al. Complications in bilateral mandibular distraction osteogenesis using internal devices. Oral Surg Oral Med Oral Pathol Oral Radiol Endod 2003;96(4):392–7.

35. Shetye PR, Warren SM, Brown D, et al. Documentation of the incidents associated with mandibular distraction: introduction of a new stratification system. Plast Reconstr Surg 2009;123:627–34.

36. Pruzansky S, Richmond J. Growth of mandible in infants with micrognathia. Am J Dis Child 1954;88:29–42.

37. Kaban LB, Moses MH, Mulliken JB. Surgical correction of hemifacial microsomia in the growing child. Plast Reconstr Surg 1988;82:9–19.

Endoscopic Skull Base Techniques for Juvenile Nasopharyngeal Angiofibroma

Adam M. Zanation, MD*, Candace A. Mitchell, BA, Austin S. Rose, MD

KEYWORDS

- Juvenile nasopharyngeal angiofibroma • Endoscopic skull base resection
- Expanded endonasal

KEY POINTS

- Juvenile nasopharyngeal angiofibroma (JNA) is a benign but locally aggressive vascular tumor that primarily affects adolescent boys. Preoperative embolization reduces intraoperative blood loss and should be done within 24 to 48 hours preoperatively.
- Preoperative angiography at the time of embolization can help to identify internal carotid artery and/or contralateral blood supply.
- The exact etiology of JNA remains unknown.
- Most JNAs can be resected via an endoscopic endonasal approach with decreased morbidity and comparable rates of blood loss and recurrence.

Key Abbreviations: Juvenile Nasopharyngeal Angiofibroma	
GW	Greater wing
ICA	Internal carotid artery
ITF	Infratemporal fossa
JNA	Juvenile nasopharyngeal angiofibroma
NP	Nasopharynx
PMF	Pterygomaxillary fossa
PPF	Pterygopalatine fossa
SPA	Sphenopalatine artery
SPF	Sphenopalatine foramen

A VIDEO ON ENDOSCOPIC SURGICAL TECHNIQUE FOR JNA ACCOMPANIES THIS ARTICLE AT http://www.oto.theclinics.com/.

Financial Disclosures/Conflict of Interest: The authors have nothing to disclose.
Department of Otolaryngology–Head & Neck Surgery, University of North Carolina School of Medicine, 170 Manning Drive, CB #7070, Chapel Hill, NC 27599-7070, USA
* Corresponding author.
E-mail address: adam_zanation@med.unc.edu

Otolaryngol Clin N Am 45 (2012) 711–730
doi:10.1016/j.otc.2012.03.008
0030-6665/12/$ – see front matter Published by Elsevier Inc.

INTRODUCTION

Juvenile nasopharyngeal angiofibroma (JNA) is a benign vascular neoplasm, the etiologic origin of which remains elusive.[1] Although typically slow growing, these nonencapsulated tumors are locally aggressive, with the potential for intracranial or intraorbital extension. JNAs typically arise from the posterolateral wall of the naso-pharynx and grow by extrusion via natural ostia. Advanced tumors often assume a dumbbell-shaped configuration, with one portion of the tumor occupying the naso-pharynx and the other portion reaching into the pterygopalatine fossa (PPF).[2] Intracra-nial extension occurs in approximately 10% to 20% of patients.[3–5] JNAs typically derive their blood supply from the ipsilateral internal maxillary artery, a branch off the external carotid artery (ECA); however, bilateral supply and communication with the internal carotid are relatively common. Wu and colleagues[6] described bilateral vascularity in 36% of patients, with ipsilateral internal carotid artery (ICA) contribution present in 10% of cases. Up to one-third of tumors have contributions from the ascending pharyngeal artery as well. As JNAs expand, they may also recruit additional blood supply from the ophthalmic and contralateral internal maxillary arteries.

JNAs are rare, representing a mere 0.5% of head and neck tumors (approximate incidence = 1:150,000)[2,4,7] and occur almost exclusively in adolescent male patients. Isolated cases exist of JNAs presenting in female patients and older men.[8,9] The most common presenting symptoms are epistaxis and progressive nasal obstruction; most patients present concurrently with both symptoms.[5] Other presenting symptoms include nasal discharge, pain, sinusitis, otologic symptoms, visual loss, facial defor-mity, facial hypesthesia, diplopia (from cranial nerve compression or from direct orbital compression), and proptosis. At the time of presentation, a red-to-purple nasal mass may be visible on gross inspection of the nasal cavity (**Fig. 1**).[10]

Workup for suspected JNA begins with in-office endoscopy, followed by radio-graphic imaging typically including both computed tomography (CT) and magnetic resonance imaging (MRI) modalities. CT scans are preferred for assessment of the extent of bony invasion (**Fig. 2**), whereas MRI provides superior visualization of the soft tissue of the tumor itself as well as of adjacent structures such as the ICA, cavernous sinus, and pituitary gland (**Fig. 3**).[10] The Holman-Miller sign, anterior bowing of the posterior maxillary wall, is usually best appreciated on axial CT scan and is considered pathognomonic for JNA. Angiography provides further confirmation of the diagnosis to allow for concurrent preoperative embolization (**Fig. 4**).[10] Biopsy confirmation of the histologic diagnosis is not performed until in the operating room,

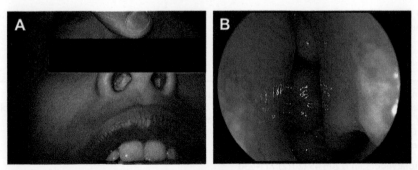

Fig. 1. (*A*) Right JNA extending anteriorly along the floor of the nose. (*B*) Endoscopic view of left JNA, extending into the nasal cavity and along the floor of the nose.

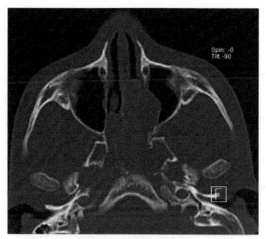

Fig. 2. Axial CT scan of left JNA filling the nasopharynx, causing bowing of the maxillary sinus and extension into the PPF.

after embolization, because of the extensive vascularity of these lesions and the potential for significant bleeding.

Surgical resection is the definitive treatment modality for JNA and is largely curative, although recurrence may occur in a minority of patients.[9] Preoperative embolization is typically performed 24 to 48 hours before scheduled surgery to decrease intraoperative bleeding risk. In the past, resections of JNA have typically been done

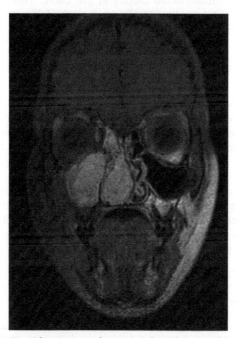

Fig. 3. A coronal MRI, T1 with contrast, shows a right-sided JNA filling the maxillary sinus and distorting the orbital floor with secondary proptosis.

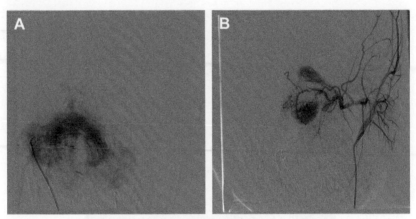

Fig. 4. (*A*) Preoperative embolization of an extensive right-sided JNA, via the right ECA and internal maxillary artery. (*B*) Preoperative embolization of left JNA.

via open approaches. However, endoscopic approaches are quickly becoming the treatment of choice. An incision-free approach obviates the risk of growth center disruption and facial asymmetry in this young population. Furthermore, evidence suggests that endoscopic techniques may decrease operative time, blood loss, and need for transfusion, although definitive data are lacking.[9] This review focuses on endoscopic techniques and outcomes for JNA. We also discuss potential future adjuncts to surgical treatment through genomic and hormonal translational research.

> PEARLS & PITFALLS: *In cases in which a JNA or other vascular sinonasal tumor is suspected, one should avoid biopsy in the clinic. This is generally best done in the operating room, usually as a part of the surgical resection, because of the risk of significant bleeding.*

PREOPERATIVE CONSIDERATIONS
Staging

Several staging systems have been proposed and modified to classify JNA, and most are based on the extent and location of the tumor. The 3 main staging systems are outlined in **Table 1**. The Radkowski system is the most widely used for JNA classification, dividing tumors into 3 distinct groups (see **Table 1**). The primary limitation of these older staging systems is that they were not designed for endoscopic approaches.

Thus, Snyderman and colleagues[11] at the University of Pittsburgh Medical Center (UPMC) published an endoscopic staging system for JNA. They note that tumor size and the extent of sinus disease are less important in predicting complete tumor removal with endonasal surgical techniques. The UPMC staging system for JNA accounts for 2 important prognostic factors:

1. Route of cranial base extension
2. Residual vascularity after embolization (often signifying the presence of internal carotid or bilateral blood supply).

Compared with other staging systems, Snyderman and colleagues[11] assert that the UPMC system provides a better prediction of immediate morbidity (including blood loss and need for multiple operations) as well as tumor recurrence (**Table 2**).

Table 1
Current staging systems for JNA

	Stage 1	Stage 2	Stage 3	Stage 4
Onerci,[45] 2006	Nose, NP, and ethmoid and sphenoid sinuses or minimal extension into PMF	Maxillary sinus, full occupation of PMF, extension to anterior cranial fossa, limited extension into ITF	Deep extension into cancellous bone at pterygoid base or body and GW sphenoid; significant lateral extension into ITF or pterygoid plate, orbital, cavernous sinus obliteration	Intracranial extension between pituitary gland and ICA, middle fossa extension, and extensive intracranial extension
Radkowski et al,[49] 1996	1a Limited to nose or NP 1b Stage 1a with extension into 1 or more sinuses	2a Minimal extension through SPF and into medial PMF 2b Full occupation of PMF, displacing posterior wall of maxilla forward, orbit erosion, displacement of maxillary artery branches 2c ITF, cheek, posterior to pterygoid plates	Erosion of skull base: 3a Minimal intracranial extension 3b Extensive intracranial extension with or without cavernous sinus	N/A
Andrews et al,[48] 1989	Limited to NP, bone destruction negligible or limited to SPF	Invading PPF or maxillary, ethmoid or sphenoid sinus with bone destruction	Invading ITF or orbit 3a No intracranial involvement 3b No extradural and parasellar involvement	Intracranial, intradural tumor 4a With cavernous sinus, pituitary, or optic chiasm infiltration 4b Without cavernous sinus, pituitary, or optic chiasm infiltration
Chandler et al,[47] 1984	Limited to NP	Extension into nasal cavity or sphenoid sinus	Tumor into antrum, ethmoid sinus, PMF, ITF, orbit, or cheek	Intracranial extension
Sessions et al,[46] 1981	1a Limited to nose and NP 1b Extension into 1 or more sinuses	2a Minimal extension into PMF 2b Full occupation of PMF with or without erosion of orbit 2c ITF with or without cheek extension	Intracranial extension	N/A

Abbreviations: GW, greater wing; ITF, infratemporal fossa; N/A, not applicable; NP, nasopharynx; PMF, pterygomaxillary fossa; SPF, sphenopalatine foramen.

Table 2	
UPMC staging system for JNA	
Stage	**UPMC Staging System**
1	Nasal cavity, medial PPF
2	Paranasal sinuses, lateral PPF; no residual vascularity
3	Skull base erosion, orbit, infratemporal fossa; residual vascularity
4	Skull base erosion, orbit, infratemporal fossa; residual vascularity
5	Intracranial extension, residual vascularity; M, medial extension; L, lateral extension

Data from Snyderman CH, Pant H, Carrau RL, et al. A new endoscopic staging system for angiofibromas. Arch Otolaryngol Head Neck Surg 2010;136(6):588–94.

Endoscopic Anatomy

As one considers an anterior endonasal approach, it is crucial to bear in mind the relative anatomic position of the origin, as well as the spread of a JNA.

JNAs typically originate in the area of the sphenopalatine artery (SPA) and in the area of the PPF. Most commonly, the presenting symptoms are epistaxis, resulting from the weeping of blood from this vascular tumor supplied by the SPAs, and nasal congestion, related to the blockage of 1 or both choanae.

Pterygopalatine fossa

It is important to understand the complete anatomic relationship of the PPF to fully appreciate complexities involved in resection of a JNA as well as to maintain vascular control during the procedure.

- The PPF is a small pyramidal space that is limited by the posterior wall of the maxilla on its anterior surface and by the pterygoid plates along its posterior surface.
- The ascending process of the palatine bone defines the medial boundary, and its lateral boundary is the pterygomaxillary fissure, a soft tissue space separating the PPF from the infratemporal fossa along a sagittal plane at the level of the inferior orbital fissure.
- The pterygomaxillary fissure transmits the internal maxillary artery from the ECA into the PPF.
- The anterior portion of the PPF contains the terminal division of the internal maxillary artery, the terminal branches being the palatine arteries, SPA, and posterior nasal septal artery. It also gives off an infraorbital artery that runs with the maxillary division of the trigeminal nerve (V2), as well as a small perforating blood supply to the soft tissue components within the PPF.
- The more posterior compartment of the PPF contains V2, the vidian nerve, and the sphenopalatine ganglion and its terminal branches. In a recent anatomic dissection published in *The Laryngoscope*,[12] all neural structures of the PPF were located posterior to the SPA and lateral to the sphenopalatine foramen. This configuration allows access to the vascular structures of the PPF when dissecting in an anterior to posterior direction from an endonasal approach without direct damage to the nerves residing in the more posterior compartment. It should be noted that the number and course of the palatine nerves, as well as the branching pattern of the SPA, are often multiple and variable, ranging from 2 to 7 branches.[13]

Understanding the relative spread outside the PPF for surgical dissection requires a comprehensive grasp of:

- Anatomy of the PPF

- JNA's origin therein
- Propensity of JNAs to spread directly through natural anatomic pathways rather than through destructive invasion

Common routes of direct extension beyond the PPF include extension into:

- The orbit via the infraorbital fissure
- Infratemporal fossa via the pterygomaxillary fissure
- Middle cranial fossa either by traveling through the infraorbital fissure to the foramen rotundum or by traveling through the foramen ovale from the infratemporal fossa
- Anterior cranial vault via direct extension through the ethmoid cavity

Tumors invading the anterior cranial vault by this last route often accumulate blood supply from the anterior and posterior ethmoid arteries and extend into the planum sphenoidale or the ethmoid roof. Occasionally, extension into the palate can be seen through the descending palatine canals. However, these very small bony channels tend to be more resistant to the direct spread of JNA than the areas aforementioned. Of note, while this tumor type usually pushes boundaries rather than directly invading them, in rare cases it can invade through the periorbita or the dura.

Infratemporal fossa
Particular anatomic considerations in the infratemporal fossa include the substantial and variable blood supply coming from multiple branches of the ICA, including the ascending pharyngeal artery and the deep temporal arterial system. In addition, within the infratemporal fossa, feeders can come from the internal carotid, as well as from the foramen lacerum. Dissection laterally into the infratemporal fossa in the coronal plane is possible via an endonasal approach but often requires an anterior medial Denker's type maxillectomy to allow for lateral access for instrumentation.

Special considerations regarding potential for skull base reconstruction
Special considerations to make while approaching the anterior cranial fossa focus on the potential need for skull base reconstruction include:

- If vascularized reconstruction is to be performed, one must bear in mind that embolization and surgical dissection often disrupts sphenopalatine blood supply to the posterior nasal septum and middle and inferior turbinates on the side of the tumor. Therefore, vascularized flaps should be considered from the contralateral side for dural reconstruction.
- If the tumor extends posteriorly into the infratemporal fossa, it can disrupt the Eustachian tube, can cause trismus, and may pick up significant blood supply from the internal carotid system. Anatomic dissections in this area require a thorough understanding of the anatomy and demand surgical dexterity to control the carotid in the carotid canal and foramen lacerum.

Pterygoid plate removal
Traversing posteriorly from the PPF, the pterygoid plates are encountered first. If the pterygoid plates are removed medially to laterally, then the muscular insertions are encountered, including the lateral pterygoid, medial pterygoid, tensor veli palatini, and levator veli palatini muscles. If the muscular attachments are dissected free and displaced laterally, this approach gives access to more posterior structures. Thus, direct access to the cartilaginous Eustachian tube is achieved, which sits between the pterygoid area and pterygoid musculature and the foramen lacerum.

Eustachian tube dissection

If the Eustachian tube is dissected from a medial to lateral plane, then the dissection follows superiorly toward its attachment at the skull base at the bony-cartilaginous Eustachian tube junction. There is an intimate relationship with the carotid canal, and the superior and posterior portions of the cartilaginous Eustachian tube are often in continuity with the inferior portion of the foramen lacerum, through which pass the carotid artery and the cervical sympathetic chain. Tumors involving this area often pick up significant blood supply from the foramen lacerum portion of the carotid artery but may also derive blood supply from the paraclival portions of the carotid. Tumors incorporating the clival portions of the carotid often have venous outflow into the clival plexus, which can be difficult to control intraoperatively.

Poststyloid parapharyngeal space

Lateral to the infratemporal fossa, behind the pterygoids, lies the poststyloid parapharyngeal space. This space transmits the carotid sheath with the carotid artery, jugular bulb, and lower cranial nerves. It is rare for a JNA to involve this area. If JNAs were to involve this area, then a combination endoscopic and lateral approach or a staged endoscopic approach should be considered.

Preoperative anatomic scrutiny

Intimate knowledge of the anatomy of the PPF as well as the surrounding anatomic spaces should be considered essential before performing resections of tumors in this area. Preoperative CT and MRI, as well as preoperative angiography, should be scrutinized by surgeons to familiarize themselves with the vascular blood supply of the tumor. In addition, these modalities allow the surgeon to assess for potential spread outside the PPF and the need to dissect critical structures such as the orbit, infratemporal fossa, or cranial vault. Posterior extension into the Eustachian tube and into the pterygoid and masticator space should alert the surgeon to a more variable blood flow with possible blood flow derived from the ICA, as well as the potential need for a combined endoscopic and open resection or staged endoscopic resection.

ENDOSCOPIC TECHNIQUES FOR JNA REMOVAL

The endoscopic endonasal techniques for removal of JNAs follow the same basic tenets of all endoscopic skull base surgery. The patient is scheduled for surgery after appropriate workup, patient selection, and patient counseling regarding risks and benefits.

Preoperative Observation and Testing

At our institution, patients with JNA are typically admitted for observation following angiography and transcatheter embolization the day before the planned operation. The femoral site is inspected and monitored. A standard array of laboratory studies are obtained as part of the preoperative workup, including a chemistry panel, complete blood cell count, coagulation panel, and a type and crossmatch for 2 units of packed red blood cells. The angiography and embolization results are then reviewed by the surgical and vascular interventional radiology teams. Steroids are administered, usually dexamethasone (Decadron) at 10 mg every 8 hours, to prevent tumor inflammation. Surgical resection is generally performed on the first or second day following embolization to minimize revascularization as well as to limit the postembolization inflammatory response.

Routine use of CT image guidance with or without MRI fusion should be considered as a standard of care for endoscopic skull base surgery. When a JNA involves both sides of the skull base and nasopharynx or has significant infratemporal fossa extension, the results of either CT angiography or magnetic resonance angiography may also be fused for better image guidance.

Basic Tenets of Removing a JNA

The 3 basic tenets (in order) of removing a JNA are:

1. Creating appropriate space in the nasal cavities to allow for a vascular dissection.
2. Maintaining vascular control.
3. Removing tumor from the more superior portions of the ventral skull base, such as the orbit and the middle and anterior cranial fossae. If there is significant vascular exposure of the ICA, significant exposure of the dura, or creation of a cerebrospinal fluid (CSF) leak, reconstruction must be considered.

Preparation for JNA Removal

Proper preoperative communication with the surgical team is paramount in management of these tumors. This includes maintaining dialogue with the anesthesiologist regarding blood loss and replacement needs as well as communication with other members of the surgical team to have hemostatic agents and Foley catheters (to place pressure on arterial bleeding) readily available in the event of significant arterial injury.

After induction of anesthesia, the patient is registered with the image guidance system. Thereafter, the operation may proceed once the surgical team and anesthesia team have a mutual understanding of the potential for significant blood loss and for complications related to orbital and intracranial structures.

JNA Debulking

- Typically, the nasal portion of the tumor must first be debulked to provide better access to the sinonasal structures.
- Debulking can be done with bipolar cautery and true-cut instrumentation.
- Occasionally, tumors are soft enough to allow use of a tissue microdebrider.

Operative Technique

- Once the inferior and middle turbinates can be defined and the choana can be visualized, a medial maxillectomy is usually performed. This involves removing the inferior turbinate and opening the entire lateral wall of the nasal cavity into the maxillary sinus.
- Sometimes, the middle turbinate must also be removed to reach the lateral ethmoid. This exposure provides direct access to the posterior wall of the maxillary sinus, which is the anterior portion of the PPF.
- The mucosa overlying the posterior wall should then be removed.
- The bone should be thinned and removed, providing direct transmaxillary access to the PPF.
- The tumor usually fills a portion of the PPF; however, it may completely fill the PPF and extend into the infratemporal fossa, superior orbital fissure, and possibly even the middle fossa.
- If there is significant extension into the ethmoid cavities or the sphenoid sinus, those areas should be resected before tackling the infratemporal fossa component. However, if there is concern for ICA involvement, it is prudent to deal with the portion coming from the ECA first.

- The basic tenet of "one bleeder at a time" during skull surgery should be respected. Most commonly, the primary vascular supply derives from the internal maxillary artery as it enters the PPF.
- Once the fibrotic pseudocapsule of the tumor can be dissected into the PPF, the internal maxillary artery can often be identified, clipped using hemoclips and bipolar cautery, and transected from the lateral edge of the PPF portion of the tumor. Such a maneuver truncates the ECA vascular feed so that the remainder of the dissection has significantly less blood loss. It should be noted, however, that certain tumors might also derive vascular supply from the lacerum portion of the ICA, as well as contralateral ECA feeders. Such collateral supply should have been evident on 4-vessel angiography performed before the surgical procedure.
- At this point, removal of the nasal portions of the tumor is complete, and the PPF portion of the tumor is likely disconnected from its blood supply.
- If the tumor has direct extension into the orbit, the infraorbital fissure may be accessed via the PPF to remove the orbital portion of the fibrotic tumor.
- If there is significant infratemporal fossa extension, a Denker's medial maxillectomy may have to be performed to allow for more lateral access, or a sublabial Caldwell-Luc type approach may be necessary if maximal lateral access is required.
- If the tumor does involve the infratemporal fossa, it is more likely to have acquired vascular supply significantly more lateral than the PPF. This possibility makes vascular dissection of the infratemporal fossa less predictable, more variable, and technically more difficult than tumors isolated to the PPF.
- Tumors involving the middle cranial fossa or anterior cranial fossa should be gently dissected out using a 2-surgeon, 4-handed technique: one surgeon dissects while a second experienced endoscopic surgeon drives the endoscope and performs any necessary retraction and suctioning.
- Usually JNAs do not invade the dura or have dural transgression; if there is skull base involvement, it is usually erosive and extradural.
- Care should be taken to identify the dissection plane between the dura and the tumor, and the tumor should be gently dissected from the cranial dura.
- If there is a CSF leak, the tumor resection should proceed; however, it is crucial to minimize blood exchange with the CSF space. Any CSF leak created should be reconstructed at the end of the procedure.
- It should be noted that JNAs with middle fossa extension occasionally acquire vascular supply from the middle meningeal artery. Similarly, tumors with anterior cranial fossa extension may have vascular supply from the anterior and posterior ethmoidal arteries. It is not unreasonable to stage portions of the resection of a JNA if there is excessive blood loss, especially for large tumors involving numerous adjacent spaces.
- The areas in which tumors demonstrate intracranial extension or involvement of the ICA are dissected in a separate setting. Such staging allows the patient and the anesthesia team to accommodate blood loss and prevents significant surgeon fatigue resulting from sequential dissection of multiple vascular areas.

Giant JNAs

Special consideration should be given to giant JNAs. A posterior septectomy is at times warranted to allow for the binostril dissection of a large tumor, especially one involving the ICAs in the clival areas. Having a common cavity in these situations, similar to that achieved in minimally invasive pituitary surgery, allows for better access and mobility for dissection and a larger reservoir for blood to collect away from the field during dissection. When considering septectomy, it must be borne in mind that a septectomy at the beginning of the procedure will destroy any potential nasoseptal flap reconstructive options. Thus, if a septal flap is expected to be necessary for reconstruction, the flap should be harvested tucked into the nasopharynx on the less-involved side. The septectomy can then be performed with the flap safely preserved for use at the end of the case.

Immediate Postoperative Care Following JNA Resection

- Once the tumor is completely resected, warm water irrigation (110°F) is copiously performed throughout the cavity.
- Any residual bleeding is controlled with bipolar cautery or pressure.
- Floseal (Baxter, Deerfield, IL, USA) is usually packed into the areas of the PPF and infratemporal fossa compounds.
- Gelfoam (Pfizer, New York, NY, USA) is then routinely laid over the Floseal, and pressure is applied using a Foley balloon for 24 hours.
- In cases of a small tumor with minimal blood loss, the patient can be monitored in a standard floor bed; however, if the patient experiences significant blood loss or for larger JNAs, it is advisable to monitor the patient in the intensive care unit (ICU) while the Foley is in place.
- The Foley is removed on postoperative day 1.
- The patient is then started on nasal saline sprays for 1 week and is transitioned to nasal saline irrigations thereafter. Routinely, the patient is discharged home on this irrigation regimen with instructions to refrain from nose blowing and strenuous activity, including instructions regarding bowel regimens in the setting of constipation.
- Any events of arterial bleeding should necessitate an endoscopy and possible repeated surgical intervention.
- If patients present with a bleed in the outpatient setting, they should be instructed to report immediately to the emergency room.

PEARLS & PITFALLS: When removing a Foley catheter used as nasal packing, deflate the balloon and leave the catheter in place for 5 minutes before complete removal. This way, the balloon can simply be reinflated for any significant epistaxis.

CSF Leak in JNA Surgery

Special consideration should be given to reconstruction if there is a CSF leak.

- Options for skull base reconstruction routinely include the use of vascularized flaps, such as the nasal septal flap.
- In these cases, the flap is then placed over the defect and is bolstered into place with SurgiSeal (Adhezion, Wyomissing, PA, USA), DuraSeal (Covidien, Mansfield, MA, USA), and absorbable packing.
- Nonabsorbable packing is then placed underneath, either in the form of a Foley balloon or in the form of finger Cotton-Merocel (Merocel, Mystic, CT, USA) packs.
- If it is a low-flow leak, packing is left in place for 3 days.
- For high-flow leaks with a leak into the cistern, packing remains in place for 7 days.
- Lumbar drainage in the postoperative period should be considered for patients with high-flow CSF leaks, usually performed for 3 days at 10 mL/h.

- If there is a significant CSF leak at the time of the operation, a postoperative head CT is performed to establish a baseline level of pneumocephalus for future comparisons.
- The patient is routinely placed in the neurologic ICU and is followed up with serial neurologic checks.
- Broader-spectrum antibiotic coverage using third- or fourth-generation cephalosporins is used while packs are in place.

Postoperative Follow-Up

- In the postoperative setting, patients undergo sinonasal endoscopy with debridements in the clinical setting at approximately 2 weeks and again at 4 to 6 weeks.
- The postoperative cavity is usually well mucosalized by 6 to 12 weeks after surgery.
- Multidisciplinary follow-up may be necessary in certain cases.
- If the patient has significant orbital involvement, postoperative follow-up with ophthalmologic examination for transient double vision may be warranted.
- If an aggressive Denker's medial maxillectomy was performed and the nasal lacrimal duct was transected sharply, postoperative transient epiphora may be expected.
- Follow-up with neurosurgical examinations may be necessary if there was significant intracranial extension or a substantial CSF leak.
- Follow-up in the first year is usually every 3 months.
- It has become our tendency routinely to obtain a postoperative MRI with contrast in the first 3 months (**Fig. 5**) if we believe we achieved a total resection, so that we have baseline imaging for future comparison to detect recurrence.
- If portions of the tumor might need to be reresected or staged, we obtain an early MRI during the immediate postoperative hospitalization for planning.

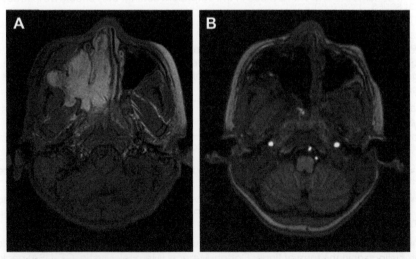

Fig. 5. (A) Axial MRI, T1 with contrast, demonstrates a large right-sided JNA before endoscopic resection. Tumor fills the right nasal passage, nasopharynx, and maxillary sinus and extends into the infratemporal fossa and between the medial and lateral pterygoid muscles. (B) Same patient as in A after endoscopic skull base resection of right JNA with complete removal of tumor radiographically.

- Future imaging studies usually consist of MRI at 1 year and clinical follow-up thereafter.
- Late recurrences are possible, and the patients are therefore followed up into adulthood.

OUTCOMES OF ENDOSCOPIC SURGERY FOR JNA

To assess the existing data on endoscopic surgery for JNA, we analyzed more than 350 endoscopic resections of JNAs as described in various case series in the past decade (**Table 3**).[8,9,14–31] The vast preponderance of these resections are described:

- Without complications (4 of 352 cases, 1.1%)
- With minimal persistent disease (12 of 352 cases, 3.4%)
- With similarly low recurrence rates (16 of 352 cases, 6.5%).

Average blood loss is nearly uniformly described as lower than that with comparable open surgical approaches, with average blood loss ranging from 168 mL, in series with only low-stage tumors, to 1500 mL, in series with high-stage (Radkowski stage IIIa or greater) tumors. Average blood loss across studies reporting this data point was 445 mL, and average length of hospital stay was 4 days. These numbers compare favorably with generally quoted numbers for open approaches; in a series by Hackman and colleagues,[9] mean blood loss in 4 patients with open approaches averaged 2500 mL (range, 450–7000 mL), and all required transfusion.

Admittedly, these data are prone to significant selection bias because endoscopic approaches tend to be favored in lower-stage disease. However, even in series such as that in the study by Nicolai and colleagues,[30] in which 17 of 46 (37%) patients who underwent endoscopic resection had disease of Andrews stage IIIa or greater (Andrews type III: tumor invading infratemporal fossa or orbital region without intracranial involvement [a] or with intracranial extradural [parasellar] involvement), no complications and no recurrent disease was reported. Of the 4 cases of persistent disease in that series, 3 were Andrews stage IIIa or greater. Overall, at least 94 (26.6%) of a total of 386 cases reviewed were documented as high-stage disease (generally Radkowski stage IIIa or greater). Even if all adverse outcomes documented were within this high-stage population (this cannot be determined through the published literature), they would constitute rates of persistent and recurrent disease of 12 of 94 (12.8%) and 23 of 94 (24.5%), respectively. With overall recurrence rates for JNA quoted at 13% to 46%,[10,32] even such high estimates of suboptimal outcomes in this high-risk population would be at least comparable, if not superior, to open approaches.

Such evaluation of the available literature, then, suggests that endoscopic approaches have the potential to be as effective and safe as traditional open approaches, even in advanced disease. Combined with the generally accepted advantages of endoscopic surgery, such as favorable cosmetic result and superior intraoperative visualization, this affirmation of the efficacy and safety of endoscopic approaches supports a shift toward endoscopic resection of even the most complicated JNAs.

ADJUNCTIVE AND ALTERNATIVE THERAPIES
Radiation Treatment

Although radiation treatment of JNA was considered to be a viable alternative to surgery for some time, involution of tumor took up to 3 years. In addition, radiation therapy carries the potential for induction of malignancy and inhibition of facial growth, important considerations in this primarily adolescent patient population. Lee and colleagues[33] performed a retrospective analysis of 27 patients who received 3000

Table 3
Endoscopic surgery for JNA: current literature

Study	Patients in Study	Endoscopic Resections	Staging System	Advanced Stage Tumors Included	Complications	Persistent Disease	Recurrences	Blood Loss (mL)	Hospital Stay (d)	Notes
Roger et al,[14] 2002	20	20	Radkowski	9	0	2	0	350	—	—
Onerci et al,[15] 2003	12	12	Radkowski	4	—	2	0	1000	—	Blood loss reported for low-stage tumors; blood loss for high-stage tumors is 1500 mL
Hoffman et al,[16] 2005	21	21	—	3	—	3	3	225	2	—
Pryor et al,[17] 2005	65	5	—	—	—	—	0	—	—	—
Tosun et al,[18] 2006	24	9	Radkowski	2	0	—	0	1 transfusion	—	—
de Brito Macedo Ferreira et al,[19] 2006	9	9	Chandler	1	0	0	0	1 patient required transfusion	8	Embolization performed average of 4.5 d preoperatively
Baradaranfar & Dabirmoghaddam,[20] 2006	105 (32 JNA)	32	Radkowski	0	—	—	2	—	—	—
Eloy et al,[21] 2007	6	6	Radkowski	0	—	—	1	575	—	—
Andrade et al,[22] 2007	12	12	Andrews	0	0	0	0	200	3	—
Yiotakis et al,[23] 2008	20	9	—	0	0	0	0	248.8	2	—
Gupta et al,[24] 2008	28	28	Radkowski	0	1 intraoperative internal maxillary artery bleed	1	0	168	—	Blood loss reported for patients who underwent preoperative embolization. For nonembolized patients, average blood loss is 360 mL
Huang et al,[25] 2009	19	19	Radkowski	5	—	—	0	—	—	—

Study								Blood loss (mL)		Comments
Bleier et al,[26] 2009	18	10	Andrews	1	0	—	1	506	3	4-d hospital stay for open resection
Midilli et al,[8] 2009	42	12	Radkowski	1	—	—	—	No transfusions required	5	5- to 7-d hospital stay for open resection
Zhou et al,[27] 2010	59	59	Radkowski	34	—	—	6	—	—	All recurrences were in patients with high-stage tumors
Hackman et al,[9] 2009	31	15	—	3	1 retro-orbital hemorrhage	—	1	280	—	—
Nicolai et al,[30] 2010	46	46	Onerci/Andrews 25	0	4	0	—	580	5	25 advanced tumors by Onerci staging; 23 by Andrews staging
Ardehali et al,[28] 2010	47	47	Radkowski	4	2 ruptures of cavernous sinus	—	9	770	3.1	Blood loss reported for patients who underwent preoperative embolization. For nonembolized patients, average blood loss is 1402.6 mL. Hospital stay for embolized patients is 1.8 d
Renkonen et al,[29] 2010	27	3	Andrews	0	—	—	0	—	—	—
Fyrmpas et al,[31] 2011	10	10	Radkowski	2	—	0	—	444	5	—
Total	548	353	—	94	12	23	—	445.57 (average)	4.01 (average)	—

Note: All reported results are for tumors resected by endoscopic approach unless otherwise specified.

to 5500 cGy as the primary treatment modality for JNA. They found that the recurrence rate for this sample was 15% at 5 years. However, at the 2-year mark, most cases still had residual tumor present before complete involution.

Cummings and colleagues[34] evaluated secondary malignancies in patients treated with external beam radiotherapy for JNA. They found secondary malignancies in 2 of the 55 cases evaluated. These were thyroid carcinoma and cutaneous basal cell carcinoma. Both cancers arose after radiation therapy and were considered a result of the treatment. At present, the treatment of choice is surgical resection. Even in the setting of recurrent disease, additional surgery should be considered before radiation. Radiotherapy should be reserved for symptomatic or progressive tumors with extensive intracranial invasion without available surgical options.

See Video demonstrating the endoscopic endonasal resection of a large right-sided JNA with extension into the right infratemporal fossa. Components within the nasal cavity, nasopharynx, maxillary sinus, sphenoid, pterygomaxillary fossa, and infratemporal fossa are addressed sequentially. Endonasal bipolar technique and use of a powered microdebrider for resection are demonstrated.

DISCUSSION OF POTENTIAL SYSTEMIC TREATMENTS

Despite recent advancements in the surgical treatment of JNA, its exact etiology and potential nonsurgical treatment has yet to be elucidated. A better understanding of this pathophysiology could certainly alter and improve overall treatment. The question of whether the initiating event in the development of these tumors occurs in the endothelium or in the stroma remains unanswered. To date, many studies have been published, but no single theory explains all the characteristics or sex predilection of this disease. Recently, Coutinho-Camillo and colleagues[1] published a comprehensive review of several proposed theories for the origin of JNA, including the possible role of steroid hormones and various growth factors and a description of associated genetic alterations.

Steroid Hormones and Nuclear Receptors

Steroid hormones have been implicated in the development of many human tumors. Breast and prostate carcinomas have hormonally-based treatments that improve overall survival and have significant tumor response rates. JNA's sex predilection and age presentation, around puberty, suggest that its development is hormone dependent. Initial studies focused on hormone imbalances, whereas others have investigated the presence of sex hormone receptors in JNA tissue. We review some of this literature later. Using electron microscopy, Kuttner and colleagues[35] described histologic and cytologic alterations in the vascular component and stromal fibroblasts in patients treated with estrogen, suggesting a direct action of the hormone within the JNA tissues. However, when compared with breast cancer controls, Johns and colleagues[36] found no evidence of the estrogen receptors (ER) in 6 JNA cases. Farag and colleagues[37] evaluated serum levels of dihydrotestosterone, testosterone, and 17β-estradiol in a small series (N = 7) of patients with JNA. Levels in this small cohort were within normal ranges, suggesting that development is not driven by abnormally elevated androgen hormone levels. Similar to prior studies,[35] this group did not detect ER in JNA tissue but did detect androgen receptors in all 7 cases studied.[37]

The influence and mechanism of action of hormones on JNA remain controversial; however, the antiandrogen drug flutamide has shown promise with significant partial response rates. Recently, Thakar and colleagues[38] published a prospective, single-arm study in which 20 patients with advanced-staged JNAs were administered flutamide orally for 6 weeks before surgical excision. In this study, pretreatment and posttreatment tumor volumes and responses were measured by MRI. The study yielded interesting results: prepubertal and postpubertal patients responded differently to hormonal therapy. Prepubertal cases had inconsistent and minimal responses, whereas 13 of 15 (87%) postpubertal cases demonstrated a partial radiographic response (mean, 16.5%; maximum, 40%). Two cases with symptomatic vision loss and optic nerve compression had visual improvement. Presurgical volume reduction correlated significantly with both serum testosterone level and postpubertal status. There were minimal side effects from this treatment. Of note, this study did not compare the histologic effects of treatment or surgical outcomes with those in a control group. The findings suggest, however, that flutamide treatment might be considered for presurgical volume reduction, symptomatic tumor compression, or advanced tumor stages. However, because no complete responses to the drug were noted, complete surgical removal remains the definitive treatment option.

Growth Factors

Angiogenesis is essential to the growth of solid tumors. Because of the highly vascular nature of JNAs, many investigators have looked at the presence of angiogenic growth factors associated with JNA. The most predominant and well-studied proangiogenic growth factor in tumor biology is vascular endothelial growth factor (VEGF). In a study by Brieger and colleagues,[39] immunohistochemical examination of 10 JNAs revealed the frequent expression of VEGF (80%) in both stromal cells and vessels. Furthermore, VEGF expression was associated with proliferation and increased vessel density, suggesting that it might promote vascularization in JNA.

Increased levels of other angiogenic factors, including basic fibroblast growth factor, transforming growth factor β_1, and VEGF receptor 2, have also been recently associated with high vessel densities in JNA.[40,41] However, the clinical and etiologic relevance of such elevations are unclear. Although many angiogenic growth factors are present in JNAs at levels that are statistically significant, it is not known if this is a causative factor or an incidental finding. In the setting of a vascular tumor, elevated vascular growth factor levels and a higher density of angiogenic proteins might be expected.

Insulin-like growth factors (IGFs)–polypeptides with a variety of functions, including stimulation of cell growth, cell division, and regulation of apoptosis–have also been implicated. Although immunohistochemical studies have revealed no expression of IGF-1 receptor in JNA tissue, Nagai and colleagues[42] reported the expression of IGF-2 in 53% of JNAs, suggesting that IGF-2 may mediate growth of these tumors via a mechanism not directly involving the IGF-1 receptor. Although several studies have associated various growth factors with JNA, a potential target in the treatment of JNA has yet to be clearly identified.

Chromosomal Abnormalities

Molecular genetic techniques and genomic analysis have begun to show preliminary evidence of amplified oncogenes and/or deleted tumor suppressor genes in JNA. There has been a preponderance of evidence that the location of genetic alterations or chromosomal loss may be directly related to the sex chromosomes (X and Y).[43,44] The presence of abnormalities on specific chromosome locations in patients with JNA, including loss of the Y chromosome, may be of great importance in revealing the pathogenesis of this disease. However, a direct causal effect of a single gene loss or overexpression is not suggested by the genetic studies. As with the potential vascular targets, there are no genetically targeted therapies for JNA currently available.

SUMMARY FOR JNA TREATMENT

Many questions remain regarding the genetics and pathogenesis of JNA. It is to be hoped that continued research efforts will lead to less invasive and more specific targeted therapies. It is clinically apparent now that resection of these tumors no longer necessitates a large, cosmetically morbid operation. Endoscopic skull base tumor surgery and endoscopic skull base reconstructions now allow for resection of advanced-staged and intracranial JNAs at experienced centers. Preliminary outcome data are promising, with trends toward decreased blood loss, length of hospital stay, morbidity, and potentially cost. The panoramic visualization of the endoscopic endonasal approach provides more precision when dissecting critical structures even when they are intracranial or within the orbit or infratemporal fossa. The tenets of vascular control, staged resections, and the possible need to convert to open surgery should be respected with endoscopic resection of JNA.

REFERENCES

1. Coutinho-Camillo CM, Brentani MM, Nagai MA. Genetic alterations in juvenile nasopharyngeal angiofibromas. Head Neck 2008;30(3):390–400.
2. Mattei TA, Nogueira GF, Ramina R. Juvenile nasopharyngeal angiofibroma with intracranial extension. Otolaryngol Head Neck Surg 2011;145(3):498–504.
3. Ungkanont K, Byers RM, Weber RS. Juvenile nasopharyngeal angiofibroma: an update of therapeutic management. Head Neck 1996;18(1):60–6.
4. Gullane PJ, Davidson J, O'Dwyer T, et al. Juvenile angiofibroma: a review of the literature and a case series report. Laryngoscope 1992;102(8):928–33.
5. Bremer JW, Neel HB 3rd, DeSanto LW, et al. Angiofibroma: treatment trends in 150 patients during 40 years. Laryngoscope 1986;96(12):1321–9.
6. Wu AW, Mowry SE, Vinuela F, et al. Bilateral vascular supply in juvenile nasopharyngeal angiofibromas. Laryngoscope 2011;121(3):639–43.
7. Batsakis JG. Tumors of the head and neck: clinical and pathological considerations. 2nd edition. Baltimore (MD): Williams & Wilkins; 1979. p. 296–300.
8. Midilli R, Karci B, Akylidiz S. Juvenile nasopharyngeal angiofibroma: analysis of 42 cases and important aspects of endoscopic approach. Int J Pediatr Otorhinolaryngol 2009;73(3):401–8.
9. Hackman T, Snyderman CH, Carrau R, et al. Juvenile nasopharyngeal angiofibroma: the expanded endonasal approach. Am J Rhinol Allergy 2009;23(1):95–9.
10. Blount A, Riley KO, Woodworth BA. Juvenile nasopharyngeal angiofibroma. Otolaryngol Clin North Am 2011;44:989–1004.
11. Snyderman CH, Pant H, Carrau RL, et al. A new endoscopic staging system for angiofibromas. Arch Otolaryngol Head Neck Surg 2010;136(6):588–94.
12. Falcon RT, Rivera-Serrano CM, Miranda JF, et al. Endoscopic endonasal dissection of the infratemporal fossa: anatomic relationships and importance of eustachian tube in the endoscopic skull base surgery. Laryngoscope 2011;121(1):31–41.
13. Hosseini SM, Razfar A, Carrau RL, et al. Endonasal transpterygoid approach to the infratemporal fossa: correlation of endoscopic and multiplanar CT anatomy. Head Neck 2012;34(3):313–20.

14. Roger G, Tran Ba Huy P, Froehlich P, et al. Exclusively endoscopic removal of juvenile nasopharyngeal angiofibroma. Arch Otolaryngol Head Neck Surg 2002;128(8):928–35.

15. Onerci TM, Yucei OT, Ogretmenoglu O. Endoscopic surgery in treatment of juvenile nasopharyngeal angiofibroma. Int J Pediatr Otorhinolaryngol 2003;67(11):1219–25.

16. Hoffman T, Bernal-Sprekelsen M, Koele W, et al. Endoscopic resection of juvenile angiofibromas—long term results. Rhinology 2005;43(4):282–9.

17. Pryor SG, Moore EJ, Kasperbauer JL. Endoscopic versus traditional approaches for excision of juvenile nasopharyngeal angiofibroma. Laryngoscope 2005; 115(7):1201–7.

18. Tosun F, Ozer C, Gerek M, et al. Surgical approaches for nasopharyngeal angiofibroma: comparative analysis and current trends. J Craniofac Surg 2006;17(1): 15–20.

19. de Brito Macedo Ferreira LM, Gomes EF, Azevedo JF, et al. Endoscopic surgery of nasopharyngeal angiofibroma. Braz J Otorhinolaryngol 2006;72(4):475–80.

20. Baradaranfar MH, Dabirmoghaddam P. Endoscopic endonasal surgery for resection of benign sinonasal tumors: experience with 105 patients. Arch Iran Med 2006;9(3):244–9.

21. Eloy P, Watelet JB, Hatert AS, et al. Endonasal endoscopic resection of juvenile nasopharyngeal angiofibroma. Rhinology 2007;45(1):24–30.

22. Andrade NA, Pinto JA, Nobrega Mde O, et al. Exclusively endoscopic surgery for juvenile nasopharyngeal angiofibroma. Otolaryngol Head Neck Surg 2007; 137(3):492–6.

23. Yiotakis I, eleftheriadou A, Davilis D, et al. Juvenile nasopharyngeal angiofibroma stages I and II: a comparative study of surgical approaches. Int J Pediatr Otorhinolaryngol 2008;72(6):793–800.

24. Gupta AK, Rajiniganth MG, Gupta AK. Endoscopic approach to juvenile nasopharyngeal angiofibroma: our experience at a tertiary care centre. J Laryngol Otol 2008;122(11):1185–9.

25. Huang J, Sacks R, Forer M. Endoscopic resection of juvenile nasopharyngeal angiofibroma. Ann Otol Rhinol Laryngol 2009;118(11):764–8.

26. Bleier BS, Kennedy DW, Palmer JN, et al. Current management of juvenile nasopharyngeal angiofibroma: a tertiary center experience 1999-2007. Am J Rhinol Allergy 2009;23(3):328–30.

27. Zhou B, Cai T, Huang Q, et al. Juvenile nasopharyngeal angiofibroma: endoscopic surgery and follow-up results. Zhonghua Er Bi Yan Hou Tou Jing Wai Ke Za Zhi 2010;45(3):180–5.

28. Ardehali MM, Samimi Ardestani SH, Yazdani N, et al. Endoscopic approach for excision of juvenile nasopharyngeal angiofibroma: complications and outcomes. Am J Otolaryngol 2010;31(5):343–9.

29. Renkonen S, Hagstrom J, Vuola J, et al. The changing surgical management of juvenile nasopharyngeal angiofibroma. Eur Arch Otorhinolaryngol 2011;268(4): 599–607.

30. Nicolai P, Villaret AB, Farina D, et al. Endoscopic surgery for juvenile angiofibroma: a critical review of indications after 46 cases. Am J Rhinol Allergy 2010;24(2):e67–72.

31. Fyrmpas G, Konstantinidis I, Constantinidis J. Endoscopic treatment of juvenile nasopharyngeal angiofibromas: our experience and review of the literature. Eur Arch Otorhinolaryngol 2012;269(2):523–9.

32. Glad H, Vainer B, Buchwald C, et al. Juvenile nasopharyngeal angiofibromas in Denmark 1981-2003: diagnosis, incidence, and treatment. Acta Otolaryngol 2007;127(3):292–9.

33. Lee JT, Chen P, Safa N, et al. The role of radiation in the treatment of advanced juvenile angiofibroma. Laryngoscope 2002;112(7 Pt 1):1213–20.

34. Cummings BJ, Blend R, Keane T. Primary radiation therapy for juvenile nasopharyngeal angiofibroma. Laryngoscope 1984;94(12 Pt 1):1599–605.

35. Kuttner K, Katekamp D, Stiller D. Hormone therapy of the juvenile angiofibroma. Arch Otorhinolaryngol 1977;214:331–8.

36. Johns ME, MacLeod RM, Cantrell RW. Estrogen receptors in nasopharyngeal angiofibromas. Laryngoscope 1980;90:628–34.

37. Farag MM, Ghanimah SE, Ragaie A, et al. Hormonal receptors in juvenile nasopharyngeal angiofibroma. Laryngoscope 1987;97:208–11.

38. Thakar A, Gupta G, Bhalla AS, et al. Adjuvant therapy with flutamide for presurgical volume reduction in juvenile nasopharyngeal angiofibroma. Head Neck 2011;33(12):1747–53.

39. Brieger J, Wierzbicka M, Sokolov M, et al. Vessel density, proliferation and immunolocalization of vascular endothelial growth factor in juvenile nasopharyngeal angiofibromas. Arch Otolaryngol Head Neck Surg 2004;130:727–31.

40. Schuon R, Brieger J, Heinrich UR, et al. Immunohistochemical analysis of growth mechanisms in juvenile angiofibromas. Eur Arch Otorhinolaryngol 2007;264: 389–94.

41. Schiff M, Gonzalez A, Ong M, et al. Juvenile nasopharyngeal angiofibroma contain an angiogenic growth factor: basic FGF. Laryngoscope 1992;102:940–5.

42. Nagai MA, Butugan O, Logullo A, et al. Expression of growth factors, protooncogenes and p53 in nasopharyngeal angiofibromas. Laryngoscope 1996;106: 190–5.

43. Schick B, Brunner C, Praetorius M, et al. First evidence of genetic imbalances in angiofibromas. Laryngoscope 2002;112:397–401.

44. Heinrich UR, Brieger C, Gosepath J, et al. Frequent chromosomal gains in recurrent juvenile nasopharyngeal angiofibroma. Cancer Genet Cytogenet 2007;175: 138–43.

45. Onerci M. Juvenile nasopharyngeal angiofibroma: a revised staging system. Rhinology 2006;44(1):39–45.

46. Sessions RB, Bryan RN, Naclerio RM, et al. Radiographic staging of juvenile angiofibroma. Head Neck Surg 1981;3(4):279–83.

47. Chandler JR, Goulding R, Moskowitz L, et al. Nasopharyngeal angiofibromas: staging and management. Ann Otol Rhinol Laryngol 1984;93(4 Pt 1):322–9.

48. Andrews JC, Fisch U, Valavanis A, et al. The surgical management of extensive nasopharyngeal angiofibromas with the infratemporal fossa approach. Laryngoscope 1989;99(4):429–37.

49. Radkowski D, McGill T, Healy GB, et al. Angiofibroma: changes in staging and treatment. Arch Otolaryngol Head Neck Surg 1996;122(2):122–9.

Index

Note: Page numbers of article titles are in **boldface** type.

Otolaryngol Clin N Am 45 (2012) 731–738
doi:10.1016/S0030-6665(12)00046-1
0030-6665/12/$ – see front matter © 2012 Elsevier Inc. All rights reserved.

oto.theclinics.com

Moving?

Make sure your subscription moves with you!

To notify us of your new address, find your **Clinics Account Number** (located on your mailing label above your name), and contact customer service at:

Email: journalscustomerservice-usa@elsevier.com

800-654-2452 (subscribers in the U.S. & Canada)
314-447-8871 (subscribers outside of the U.S. & Canada)

Fax number: 314-447-8029

Elsevier Health Sciences Division
Subscription Customer Service
3251 Riverport Lane
Maryland Heights, MO 63043

*To ensure uninterrupted delivery of your subscription, please notify us at least 4 weeks in advance of move.

Printed and bound by CPI Group (UK) Ltd, Croydon, CR0 4YY

03/10/2024

01040457-0017